Pocket Guide for the Textbook of Pharmacotherapy for Child and Adolescent Psychiatric Disorders

Pocket Guide for the Textbook of Pharmacotherapy for Child and Adolescent Psychiatric Disorders

David R. Rosenberg, M.D.
John Holttum, M.D.
Neal Ryan, M.D.
Samuel Gershon, M.D.

BRUNNER/MAZEL
· Taylor & Francis Group

USA	Publishing Office:	Taylor & Francis 325 Chestnut Street, Suite 8 Philadelphia, PA 19106 Tel: (215) 625-8900 Fax: (215) 625-2940
	Distribution Center:	Taylor & Francis 47 Runway Road, Suite G Levittown, PA 19057 Tel: (215) 269-0400 Fax: (215) 269-0363
UK		Taylor & Francis Ltd. 1 Gunpowder Square London EC4A 3DE Tel: 071 405 2237 Fax: 071 831 2035

POCKET GUIDE FOR THE TEXTBOOK OF PHARMACOTHERAPY FOR CHILD AND ADOLESCENT PSYCHIATRIC DISORDERS

3 4 5 6 7 8 9 0   E B E B   9 0 9

This book was set in New Century Schoolbook. The editor was Heather Worley. Cover design by Michelle Fleitz.

A CIP catalog record for this book is available from the British Library.
⊗ The paper in this publication meets the requirements of the ANSI Standard Z39.48-1984 (Permanence of Paper)

Library of Congress Cataloging-in-Publication Data

Pocket guide for the Textbook of pharmacotherapy for child and
    adolescent psychiatric disorders / David R. Rosenberg ... [et al.].
        p.   cm.

    1. Pediatric psychopharmacology.   I. Rosenberg, David R.
    II. Rosenberg, David R. Textbook of pharmacotherapy for child and
    adolescent psychiatric disorders.
        [DNLM: 1. Mental Disorders—drug therapy—handbooks.   2. Mental
    Disorders—in infancy & childhood—handbooks.   3. Mental Disorders—
    in adolescence—handbooks.   4. Psychotropic Drugs—therapeutic use—
    handbooks.   QV 39 P7385 1997]
    RJ504.7.P63   1997
    618.92'8918—dc21
    DNLM / DLC
    for Library of Congress   97-33193
                                                                              CIP

ISBN 0-87630-871-X(paper)

Contents

Chapter

C h a p t e r   1

Introduction

In the preface to this handbook's parent volume, *Textbook of Pharmacotherapy for Child and Adolescent Psychiatric Disorders*, the authors stated as a main purpose to provide "a practical guide to the use of modern psychiatric drugs in patients age 18 and under." Great effort went into making certain the *Textbook* would be reader-friendly, and we have received very positive feedback not only from psychiatrists, but psychologists, social workers, therapists, nursing staff and students, medical students and residents, pediatricians, and family practitioners. We are delighted that the *Textbook* has been so well received, but with 554 pages and over 1,400 references, it may have fallen short of practicality. In truth, the original project was meant to be much more like what the reader is now holding—a handbook appropriate for quick reference in both inpatient and outpatient settings, and accessible to any professional involved in the mental health care of young people.

Only during the evolution of the *Textbook* did it become apparent that any condensed summary of the field ran the risk of becoming dangerously misleading. It is the nature of child and adolescent psychopharmacology that the needs of the patients outrun the state of the art. Clinical trials of medications in children are more expensive, draw from a much smaller subject population, and are complicated by ethical and health-related risks not encountered in comparable studies of adult psychiatric patients. Practitioners are sometimes forced to accept as established, treatments that are in reality only extrapolations of adult therapies. As discussed in Chapter 2, children are not (pharmacologically speaking) merely small adults.

The rational practice of psychopharmacology should obviously be based on scientifically controlled studies. Unfortunately, once the clinician gets away from the best-studied handful of child and adolescent disorders (e.g., obsessive-compulsive disorder and attention-deficit/hyperactivity disorder) there are very few or no definitive acute studies. Furthermore, nowhere in the field of pediatric psychopharmacology are there studies that give clear answers to questions about long-term treatment for prevention of relapse or recurrence. In light of this, the rational psychopharmacologist has been given the choice of either adopting a totally nihilistic approach by deciding that he/she knows too little to prescribe psychiatric medication for children at all (an approach the authors do not find inviting), or forging ahead by extending the data from open clinical trails, anecdotal reports, and perhaps controlled trials in adults to make the best possible decisions.

On a positive note, this disconcerting lack of controlled data for child psychopharmacology is likely to improve over time. Recent efforts by the Food and Drug Administration (FDA) to work with the pharmaceutical industry to support more studies in children and adolescents will be responsible for much of the improvement. In addition, the American Psychiatric Association and the American Academy of Child and Adolescent Psychiatry are working with clinicians to gather a large naturalistic database on clinical practice which should provide a tremendous amount of uncontrolled data useful for examining those questions which are not amenable to controlled study. Against this background it becomes obvious that a thorough understanding of pediatric psychopharmacology requires not only mastery of current practices, but full knowledge of the research bases for those practices, including the astounding lack of definitive research in most areas. Therefore, in the *Textbook*, brevity was ultimately sacrificed for scientific accuracy and completeness. In this regard, we are pleased that it is now being used as core material for several graduate and postgraduate courses in child and adolescent psychopharmacology.

However, our original aim, that of producing a quick reference handbook, did not disappear. In fact, some readers of the *Textbook* have virtually demanded a companion pocket guide to serve that purpose, a demand which has now been met in this *Pocket Guide for the Textbook of Pharmacotherapy for Child and Adolescent Psychiatric Disorders*. In this volume, readers will find the "bottom line" from each of the *Textbook* chapters. Clinical indications, contraindications, dosage guidelines, side effects and their management, common drug interactions, and most of the tables from the *Textbook* have all been retained and updated, while the comprehensive critical review of psychopharmacology has largely been omitted. For this reason, the *Guide* is not intended to be used as a clinician's sole resource for prescribing practices, but as a portable companion to the *Textbook*, suitable for "quick looks" and *in situ* decision making.

For example, in the case of psychostimulants, the reader will find the practical information required to make day-to-day prescribing decisions in the *Guide*, but should also realize that this is one of the few areas in which controlled studies have established specific indications, outcome measures, pharmacokinetics, and dose/response relationships for patients under 18 years of age. Review of that research background can be found in the *Textbook*. Similarly, although the *Guide* states that monoamine oxidase inhibitors (MAOIs) have limited use in current practice, the clinician would be remiss if he did not also review the many clinical successes documented in past research on MAOIs. In the *Textbook*, one would discover the clinical potential of future compounds with a more favorable risk profile (such as moclobemide) in the treatment of attention-deficit/hyperactivity disorder (ADHD), anxiety disorders, and adolescent depression.

How to Use This Guide

Most chapters presuppose that the clinician has performed a thorough diagnostic formulation of the case in question. It is also assumed that conservative treatment measures have been undertaken in the forms of psychotherapy, environmental structuring, parent education and training, and behavioral therapy. Where appropriate, psychometric testing, medical evaluation, and neurological consultations will have been obtained before the *Guide* becomes useful. In other words, a comprehensive diagnostic assessment must be completed and all available non-pharmacologic interventions must be tried before treatment with a medication is considered. It is at this point that the clinician can accurately assess the risk/benefit profile of a particular pharmacologic therapy and communicate that assessment to the family.

The *Guide* further assumes that the clinician possesses a working knowledge of the classes of medication available for the treatment of psychiatric illness. For this reason, chapters are not organized by diagnosis, but by classes of medication. For example, once it has been decided that a heterocyclic antidepressant might be helpful, then review of Chapter 4 (Tricyclic Antidepressants) will provide the needed guidelines for selecting a specific compound, determining dosage, and scheduling follow-up examinations. If there is uncertainty regarding which medication classes can be used to treat a specific diagnosis or symptom, we advise using the index to locate treatment options for that condition. For the treatment of "anxiety" pertinent entries can be found in Chapter 4 (Tricyclic Antidepressants), Chapter 5 (Novel Antidepressants), Chapter 6 (MAOIs), Chapter 10 (Anxiolytics and Sedatives), and Chapter 11 (Adrenergic Agents).

Recent Developments

The authors have attempted to update the *Guide* to include all significant research findings available since the publication of the *Textbook*, literally up until the day the manuscript for each chapter was submitted. Nevertheless, time has passed between submission and publication and there are several new developments which bear mentioning. In the management of ADHD, for instance, newer products such as Adderall and guanfacine (Tenex) have seen greater acceptance, while two veteran treatments, pemoline (Cylert) and clonidine (Catapres), have lost some favor.

Adderall is a mixture of four amphetamine and dextroamphetamine salts previously marketed for weight loss as Obetrol. The positive reception of Adderall is at this point based on data from the pharmaceutical company and on anecdotal reports. No independent controlled trials or long-term reviews

4

of side effects have been published as of this writing. However, it should be noted that during the brief withdrawal of the drug by the FDA (for technical reasons not related to safety) there was a surprising outcry from adults with ADHD and parents of children with ADHD who had been doing well on the medication. Clinicians might find it enlightening to monitor public opinion on such matters via the Internet. As of October, 1996, 34 million households in the United States had access to the Internet, corresponding to an incredible 35% of Americans, based on U.S. Census Bureau estimates. Even more remarkable is the fact that this figure has been doubling annually since 1988. Active support groups for patients and parents coping with ADHD, Tourette's disorder, depression, bipolar disorder, and a variety of other issues are maintained through Internet newsgroups. And there is now a plethora of World Wide Web sites offering mental health information to the public and to clinicians. It has become necessary for physicians to be conversant in this relatively new form of information distribution, as it greatly affects the opinions and perceptions of their clients.

Recent concern over the safety of clonidine was sparked by a report of sudden death in three children taking clonidine and methylphenidate.[1] However, it should be noted that none of these deaths could be directly linked to clonidine. One child had no detectable clonidine or methylphenidate in post-mortem blood analysis, the second had extensive fibrotic scarring of the heart thought to be congenital, and the third died after an intentional overdose of fluoxetine. Nevertheless, the need for close cardiac monitoring, especially early in treatment when previously unidentified congenital abnormalities might be uncovered, is underscored by this report.

Similarly, concern about the safety of pemoline was raised when a 14-year-old boy died abruptly of hepatic failure after taking the medication for 16 months.[2] This is the third report of fatal pemoline-induced liver failure. Whether or not liver function tests were monitored in this case, and whether or not closer monitoring would have altered the course, are unknown.

In the wake of concern about clonidine, guanfacine has emerged as a probable replacement for use in aggressive, hyperactive children, and particularly for children with both ADHD and Tourette's disorder. Also an alpha-2 adrenergic agonist, guanfacine causes less sedation and purportedly fewer cardiac side effects than clonidine. Most available data on guanfacine treatment are from open studies, but reports have so far been favorable.

Finally, research continues to find safer and more effective antipsychotic agents. Risperidone is mentioned in Chapter 7, and has seen some success in open trials for psychosis in children and adolescents. However, it has also been associated with substantial side effects in that population, including sedation, weight gain, and galactorrhea.[3,4] Olanzapine is a newer antipsychotic, chemically related to clozapine, which has seen success in pre-clinical trials, but is virtually untried in children and adolescents. This agent is of interest because like clozapine, it shows high affinity for dopamine type-4 and $5HT_2$ receptors, and because unlike clozapine, no cases of agranulocytosis have been reported to date.

By the time the reader sees this *Guide*, some of it will be outdated. The authors choose to view this as a positive trend. For the first time in the history of child and adolescent psychopharmacology things seem to be moving rapidly. It is the authors' wish that this book will provide the practical guidance necessary to safely and effectively prescribe medication (when medication is deemed necessary) for child and adolescent psychiatric disorders, but it cannot be used as a cookbook, and it certainly does not comprise the last words on the subject. The practice of pediatric psychopharmacology is itself in adolescence, necessitating that each practitioner participate in and contribute to the growth of our understanding of how best to serve these children.

References

1. Maloney, M.J., Schwam, J.S. (1996). Clonidine and sudden death [letter]. *Pediatrics, 6*, 1176–1177.
2. Berkovitch, M., Pope, E., Phillips, J., et al. (1995). Pemoline-associated fulminant liver failure: Testing the evidence for causation. *Clin Pharmacol Ther, 57*, 696–698.
3. Hardan, A., Johnson, K., Johnson, C., et al. (1996). Case study:

Risperidone treatment of children and adolescents with developmental disorders. *J Am Acad Child Adolesc Psychiatry*, *35*, 1551–1556.

4. Lombroso, P.J., Scahill, L., King, R.A., et al. (1995). Risperidone treatment of children and adolescents with chronic tic disorders: a preliminary report. *J Am Acad Child Adolesc Psychiatry*, *34*, 1147–1152.

Characteristics of Drug Disposition during Childhood

Robert A. Branch, M.D.*

$\mathbf{A}$ child is not simply a small adult and so will have different pharmacokinetics (drug concentration at the effector site) and pharmacodynamics (drug action at the effector site and end response). Normal maturation results in changes in the physiologic determinants of drug disposition.

Regardless of the age of a child receiving a drug, the dispositional characteristics of the drug will depend on the interaction between the physicochemical properties of the drug and the physiologic process in the patient. Physical properties of the drug include molecular size, charge, pK_a or ionic disassociation constant, and lipid solubility. These factors will determine the drug's distribution, as well as the route of elimination. In general, water-soluble drugs have a small volume of distribution and can be eliminated unchanged in urine, whereas lipid-soluble drugs have a large volume of distribution and require metabolism to more water-soluble moieties prior to elimination.

Volume of Distribution (V_d)

The apparent volume of distribution is defined as the volume into which a drug distributes in the body when at equilibrium, and is related to the pool from which the drug concentration is measured. This theoretical concept reflects the partitioning

---

*Professor of Medicine and Director of the Center for Clinical Pharmacology at the University of Pittsburgh Medical Center.

of the drug among the physiologic compartments in the body.

Apart from the newborn infant, the volume of distribution is approximately linear with body weight. Thus, it is rational and common practice to modify initial loading-dose regimens to achieve a given initial plasma concentration rapidly by factoring in weight.

Protein Binding

Most drugs in plasma are reversibly bound to proteins, with acidic drugs binding predominantly to albumin and basic drugs to alpha-1-acid glycoprotein. Only unbound drug is capable of evoking a pharmacologic response. In general, serum albumin concentrations do not change from early childhood concentrations. The situation for alpha-1-acid glycoprotein is more complex. Higher concentrations of this acute-phase–acting protein are found in children, and this increase has been observed to increase the protein binding of basic psychotropic drugs, such as haloperidol, which results in reduced free-drug concentrations.[1] Intercurrent infections and physical stress are common in children and may be associated with further rises in the concentration of this protein. This would be anticipated to induce a decrease in free-drug concentration and a reduced pharmacodynamic response. In addition to influencing drug distribution, changes in protein binding can influence drug elimination. An increase in the free fraction of a drug in the blood can lead to an increase in the amount of drug available to the drug-metabolizing enzymes, and, therefore, to an increase in the total clearance of some drugs.

Drug Half-Life

Age-related changes in distribution due either to small body mass or to altered drug binding can be expected to influence a drug's half-life $(t_{1/2})$ independently of factors influencing drug elimination, which depends on both the blood clearance and the apparent volume of distribution. The smaller the child, the smaller will be the volume of distribution and the shorter the half-life. Therefore, a drug with a narrow therapeutic window (or withdrawal side effects) is likely to require more frequent dosing intervals for a child.

Drug Elimination and Clearance

Drug elimination is defined as the irreversible loss of a drug from the site of measurement; this includes both metabolism and excretion. Clearance (Cl) relates drug concentration to the rate of elimination to provide a measure of the efficiency of the elimination process. Total or systemic plasma clearance is a measure of the amount of plasma cleared of drug per unit time. This measure can be obtained from measurements of drug concentration in plasma after bolus doses or at steady state.

When the rate of elimination is proportional to the amount of drug present, it is a first-order process. Under first-order conditions, the clearance of a drug is constant over a range of concentrations. Not all drugs undergo first-order kinetics, however; in some instances, dose-dependent or zero-order elimination occurs as a result of the saturation of an energy-requiring process. Clearance in these cases is nonlinear and will vary depending on the achieved concentration of drug. For a drug with first-order kinetics, dosing increments can be expected to be associated with proportionate increases in steady-state concentrations; for a drug with zero-order kinetics, dosing increments result in exponential increases in steady-state concentrations for equal dose increments.[2]

The two major routes of elimination for most drugs are renal excretion and biotransformation, although pulmonary exhalation or direct secretion to bile can be a major route for certain drugs.

Renal excretion is related closely to measures of the glomerular filtration rate (GFR), such as creatinine clearance or even serum creatinine concentrations. In the neonatal period the GFR is low in proportion to body weight or surface area for up to six months postnatally, but thereafter meets total body requirements by more nearly reflecting surface area rather than body weight.

Biotransformation is a much more variable process.[3,4] The 10-fold to 100-fold intersubject variation for most metabolic routes in adults is reflected by an equivalent extent of variation in childhood. This wide variation is most dramatically illustrated for drugs (including many psychotropic drugs) that exhibit a genetic polymorphism of metabolic clearance due to the presence or absence of cytochrome P-4502D6.[5] Considering children at various ages, for drugs with first-order kinetics, the dose required to achieve a given steady-state plasma concentration is not well predicted by age or weight. Even the common practice of normalizing by surface area tends to result in lower plasma concentrations than those anticipated from predictions based on adults, implying that metabolic clearance is more efficient in children than would be expected in adults, using conventional normalizing approaches. Psychotropics for which this is important include carbamazepine, haloperidol, and desipramine.

Given the complexity of drug metabolism, each drug must be considered as a unique entity.

References

1. Schley, J., Muller-Oerlinghausen, B. (1983). The binding of chemically different psychotropic drugs to alpha-1-acid glycoprotein. *Pharmacopsychiatria*, *16*, 82–85.
2. Rane, A., Hojer, B., Wilson, J.T. (1976). Kinetics of carbamazepine into its 10, 11 episode metabolism in children. *Clin Pharmacol Ther*, *19*, 276–279.
3. Svensmark, O., Buchthal, F. (1964). Diphenylhydantoin and phenobarbital. Serum levels in children. *Am J Dis Child*, *108*, 82–87.
4. Gualtieri, C.T., Golden, R., Evans, R.W., Hicks, R.E. (1984). Blood level measurement of psychoactive drugs in pediatric psychiatry. *Ther Drug Monitor*, *6*, 127–141.
5. Jacqz, E., Hall, S., Branch, R.A. (1986). Genetically determined polymorphisms in oxidative drug metabolism. *Hepatology*, *6*, 1020–1032.

C h a p t e r   3

Psychostimulants

The psychostimulants primarily methylphenidate (Ritalin), dextroamphetamine sulfate (Dexedrine), and magnesium pemoline (Cylert) are the most commonly prescribed medications in all of child psychiatry. An estimated 2% of school-age children receive stimulant medication for attention-deficit/hyperactivity disorder (ADHD) symptoms.[1] These medications, which have a remarkably benign side-effect profile, have demonstrated efficacy in the treatment of disorders such as ADHD, a disorder with marked functional impairment and long-term morbidity for the child and family. There is no evidence that the use of prescribed stimulant medication results in the increased use or abuse of, or dependence on and addiction to the stimulants themselves. When used effectively, the stimulants are beneficial, safe, and cost-effective in decreasing hyperactivity, distractibility, impulsivity, and fidgetiness, and in increasing attention span. State-dependent learning is not a problem when stimulants are used. Cognitive sequelae of ADHD may respond optimally to more modest doses of these medications, while behavioral symptoms may require larger doses.[2]

Chemical Properties

For the chemical properties of the psychostimulants, see Table 3.1.

The stimulants are sympathomimetic amines that, when administered orally, are absorbed from the gastrointestinal (GI) tract and cross the blood–brain barrier.[3] The onset of action for

Table 3.1

Pharmacokinetics of Central Nervous System (CNS) Stimulants in Children and Adolescents

Generic Name (Brand Name)	Onset of Action	Peak Plasma Concentration	Plasma Half-Life	Metabolism and Excretion	Comments
Methylphenidate (Ritalin)	30–60 minutes, up to 3 hours for SR*	1–2 hours, 4–5 hours for SR*	1–2 hours	Metabolized by hepatic microsomal enzymes	Drug concentrations higher in brain than in blood
Dextroamphetamine sulfate (Dexedrine)	30–60 minutes, 1–2 hours for spansule	2 hours, 8–10 hours for spansule	6–8 hours	Partly metabolized by liver and partly excreted unchanged in urine	Excretion increased by acidification of urine, decreased by alkalinization. Develops high concentration in brain
Magnesium pemoline (Cylert)	variable, acute, and delayed effects	2–4 hours	8–12 hours	Metabolized 60% by the liver and excreted 40% unchanged in urine	Without significant sympathomimetic activity, half-life increased with chronic administration

*Sustained-release.

methylphenidate and dextroamphetamine is observed within 20 to 60 minutes, with a three- to six-hour duration of action. Stimulants exert their maximal effect on the target symptoms of ADHD, including hyperactivity, distractibility, inattentiveness, impulsivity, and fidgetiness. Sustained-release methylphenidate's onset of action can be delayed for as long as three hours, with a shorter duration of action and significantly more day-to-day variability than two daily doses of regular methylphenidate, given in the morning and early afternoon. Sustained-release dextroamphetamine and standard pemoline produce more consistent absorption and distribution than sustained-release methylphenidate.

Indications

See Table 3.2.

ADHD Children and Adolescents

Over 600,000 children per year are treated with psychostimulants for ADHD symptoms.[3] Until recently,

Table 3.2

Indications for CNS Stimulants in Childhood and Adolescent Psychiatry

---

FDA-Approved Indications:
- ADHD in childhood and adolescence
- Narcolepsy (methylphenidate and dextroamphetamine)
- Exogenous obesity (dextroamphetamine)

Possible Indications:
- ADHD in preschool children
- Undifferentiated attention-deficit disorder
- ADHD in intellectually subaverage children and adolescents
- ADHD symptoms in children and adolescents with Fragile X syndrome
- ADHD symptoms in children and adolescents with PDD (autism)
- ADHD symptoms in children and adolescents with head trauma and/or organic brain disease
- ADHD in children and/or adolescents with tic disorders (i.e., Tourette's syndrome)
- Potentiation of narcotic analgesia

---

stimulant medications were predominantly prescribed to children 6 to 10 years of age, and were often discontinued during adolescence. Subsequent investigation, however, has revealed that ADHD symptoms not uncommonly do persist into adolescence and adulthood.[4,5] Moreover, stimulants have been found to be effective in treating ADHD symptoms throughout life. Although nearly one million persons with ADHD have been treated with stimulants, they frequently are not prescribed correctly. Clinical efficacy has been demonstrated for reducing hyperactivity and distractibility, and for improving a child's social interaction skills, motivation for task performance, and academic achievement, by decreasing the interfering behaviors associated with ADHD. Stimulant-induced learning does not appear to be state-dependent, however, so that allowing ADHD children to go on medication-free holidays is not likely to result in either short- or long-term disruption of learning. In contrast to adults, children rarely experience mood elevations or euphoric effects when taking stimulants, although they may precipitate a worsening of mood and irritability. Stimulants are, therefore, not recommended for treating dysthymia or depression in children or adolescents, as they sometimes are in adult depression. Finally, it is important to emphasize that before initiating a stimulant trial, behavioral interventions, such as social skills training, problem-solving skills, behavioral modification, and family therapy, should be tried. If these are not sufficiently effective, then stimulant medications can be used. To date, there have been no studies of children on stimulants over several years to determine the long-term effects of these medications as the children progress into adulthood. Since frequently neither stimulant medication nor behavioral therapy alone is adequate to control ADHD symptoms, a combination of both modalities is most often the treatment of choice. When a multimodality approach is used in the treatment of ADHD, the likelihood of a good clinical outcome is increased. On the other hand, children who do not receive proper treatment are at significantly increased risk of having Axis I and II diagnoses, such as substance abuse and antisocial personality disorder.

Attention-Deficit/Hyperactivity Disorder with Tic Disorders (Tourette's Syndrome)

Most authorities recommend against using stimulants in children and adolescents with tic disorders. Stimulants can exacerbate preexisting motor tics or precipitate their de novo onset, including the tics characteristic of Tourette's syndrome. Most neuropsychiatrists instead recommend antipsychotics, clonidine, antidepressants, or clonazepam. Simple motor tics are, however, not infrequently seen in patients treated with stimulants, and their onset may not mandate that stimulant medication be discontinued. If there has been a significant reduction in the patient's behavioral problems, and the tics do not interfere with the child's functioning or concern parents or teachers, stimulant use may be continued, with close monitoring. The parents and child should be informed that simple tics, such as the "bunny rabbit nose," may go away with time and/or be nonproblematic. The subsequent development of additional tic behavior and/or coprolalia usually requires that the stimulant be discontinued. When a child develops outright Tourette's syndrome, the stimulants should be discontinued immediately, and the child's parents advised to inform any other clinician with whom they are in contact that the child should not receive stimulant medication. Stimulants are not, however, absolutely contraindicated in a child with a family history of Tourette's syndrome or other tic disorders. The child should be monitored very closely for tics while on stimulants, and if they develop, the stimulant should be stopped.

Narcolepsy

Narcolepsy is a disorder in which the person suffers from excessive daytime sleepiness with sudden-onset rapid-eye-movement (REM) sleep attacks, and it is most commonly diagnosed during the second decade of life.[6] Behavioral and educational interventions are usually tried first. If these methods are inadequate, particularly if the child is falling asleep in school, methylphenidate and dextroamphetamine can often ameliorate the sleep problems. Dosages of both methylphenidate and dextroamphetamine of 20 to 200 mg/day in divided doses are required. Tolerance often develops, however, underscoring the importance of continuing to implement behavioral and educational interventions. Indeed, this may minimize the development of tolerance. It is important to point out that cataplectic attacks are often refractory to treatment with stimulants. The tricyclic antidepressants (e.g., imipramine, 75 to 150 mg/day) are useful in some patients with cataplexy (see Chapter 4). Monoamine oxidase inhibitors, such as phenelzine (30 to 75 mg/day), have also been effective in treating sleep attacks of narcolepsy, but are ineffective in treating cataplexy (see Chapter 6).

Exogenous Obesity

The *Physicians' Desk Reference* lists dextroamphetamine sulfate as an established treatment for use as a short-term weight-reduction treatment for patients who have failed alternative therapy.[7] Other stimulants have been used to inhibit appetite, but tolerance to their anorectic effects often develops within two weeks, a duration of benefits that is obviously too short for them to be of value in weight-loss programs.

Reduction of Narcotic Analgesic Needs and Narcotic-Induced Side Effects

The addition of stimulants has been found to be useful in adult patients with severe cancer pain who require very high doses of narcotics that result in problematic sedation.[8] Dextroamphetamine in doses of 5 to 20 mg/day has been found to be effective in lowering the narcotic dosage requirements and resulting side effects. The dosage needs to be adjusted based on the patient's needs, when the pain is worst, and when it is critical that the patient be as alert as possible. Dextroamphetamine can be given either in a single early-morning dose or in divided doses, depending on the patient's needs.

Contraindications

See Table 3.3.

Stimulants are contraindicated when the patient is psychotic or has a history of psychosis, since they can induce a psychosis or exacerbate a preexisting one.[3,7] As stimulants cross the placenta, they should be avoided during pregnancy. Before initiating a stimulant trial, it is important to screen for the

Table 3.3

Stimulant Contraindications

Absolute
• None
Relative:

• Psychosis
   • Pregnancy
   • History of substance abuse in patient and/or family
   • Tic disorders (Tourette's syndrome) in child and/or family
   • History of adverse reaction to stimulants
   • Height/growth retardation
   • Cardiac/blood pressure anomalies
   • Impaired liver functioning (magnesium pemoline)
   • Patient being treated with MAOI (infrequent in children and adolescents)

presence of tics (Tourette's syndrome) in both the child and the family. As with any medication, stimulants should not be used for children and adolescents who have a history of adverse reactions to their use. Recent clinical investigation has demonstrated that stimulant use does not result in a significant decrease in the ultimate height of most children, although it is common to observe a reduction in weight gain.[9,10] Stimulants should not be prescribed for children with baseline hypertension and/or tachycardia. When tachycardia and/or hypertension occurs after the initiation of a stimulant trial, the effects on pulse and blood pressure are not usually clinically significant, and often do not require that the medication be discontinued. Additional investigation, including electrocardiography (ECG) and/or cardiology consultation, is recommended, however. Impaired liver functioning has been observed only with the use of pemoline. This complication does not always remit upon discontinuation of the drug so it is essential that liver function be checked in all children for whom pemoline is being considered. If baseline liver function tests (LFTs) are abnormal, pemoline should not be prescribed. Stimulants should not be prescribed within one week to 10 days of the discontinuation of a monoamine oxidase inhibitor (MAOI). There is no increased frequency of seizures with the use of stimulants.

Side Effects

See Table 3.4.

Insomnia, decreased appetite, irritability, dysphoria, and increased crying are frequent short-term side effects experienced by children receiving stimulant medications. Abdominal pain is a frequent complaint of children while initially on stimulants, but usually disappears with time. However, LFTs must be checked in children receiving pemoline to rule out a chemical hepatitis. Decreased cognitive ability is typically not observed on standard doses of stimulants (e.g., methylphenidate doses between 0.3 mg/kg/day and 0.69 mg/kg/day) and is only seen with high doses of these medications (e.g., methylphenidate

Table 3.4

Stimulant Side Effects

Common:
• Insomnia
• Decreased appetite
• Gastrointestinal pain
• Irritability
• Increased heart rate (clinically insignificant)
• Paradoxical worsening of behavior
Uncommon:
• Psychosis
• Sadness/isolation
• Major depressive episodes
• Cognitive impairment
• Growth retardation
• Tic disorders (i.e., Tourette's syndrome)
• Increased heart rate (clinically significant)
• Impaired liver functioning (pemoline only)
• Increased blood pressure
• Dizziness, lethargy, fatigue
• Nausea, constipation
• Rash/hives
• Hyperacusis
• Formication
• Necrotizing angiitis brain (IV amphetamine)

doses greater than 1 mg/kg/day). One third of children show increased hyperactivity on stimulants, which has been referred to as "behavioral rebound." To help decrease rebound observed in children, the clinician can decrease the lunchtime or early afternoon dose of the stimulant medication. Alternatively, the clinician can lower the dose to a previously tolerated dose where rebound was not observed. Motor tics or Tourette's syndrome are uncommon but potentially severe and debilitating side effect. Growth suppression is a potential side effect. There is no evidence that stimulants lower the seizure threshold or, when prescribed correctly, result in increased recreational or prescription drug use or abuse. Very rare side effects include nausea and vomiting, constipation, dizziness, lethargy, fatigue, nightmares, anxiety, rash/hives, hyperacusis, formication, fearfulness, and necrotizing angiitis, which results from intravenous (IV) amphetamine abuse.

Drug Interactions

See Tables 3.5 and 3.6.

Clinical Practice

For the dosing and administration of specific agents, see Table 3.7.

Prior to initiating treatment with stimulants, children and adolescents should have a physical examination in which heart rate, blood pressure, height, and weight are measured. The clinician should also perform a baseline screen for abnormal involuntary movements, including tics in the child and family. A pregnancy test should be performed in all female patients of child-bearing age since these medications generally should not be prescribed during pregnancy. When pemoline is administered, LFTs are required and should be drawn every six months while the child is receiving the medication. At each dose increase, blood pressure, pulse, height, and weight should be checked. Height and weight should be recorded at regular three- to four-month intervals once the child is on a stable dose of medication. At each visit, the child should be monitored for evidence of abnormal movements.

Table 3.5

Methylphenidate Drug Interactions

Inhibits Metabolism of:
• Anticoagulants (i.e., warfarin [Coumadin])
• Anticonvulsants (phenobarbital, phenytoin [Dilantin], primidone [Mysoline])
• Phenylbutazone (Butazolidin)
• Heterocyclic antidepressants (i.e., amitriptyline, Elavil)
Decreases Hypotensive Effect of:
• Guanethidine
In Combination with Imipramine can Cause:
• Confusion
• Mood lability
• Aggression
• Agitation
• Psychosis
Potentiates Effect of:
• All sympathomimetic medications (i.e., ephedrine)
• Recreational stimulants (cocaine)
Metabolism is Slowed by:
• MAOIs

Methylphenidate (Ritalin)

Methylphenidate (Ritalin), one of the safest medications in psychiatry, is the drug of choice in the treatment of ADHD. It is effective in 70 to 80% of children and adolescents. It has a quick onset of action and a very short half-life (see Table 3.1).

Methylphenidate-SR, 20 mg, can take up to three hours to exert an effect. In theory, 20 mg of sustained-release methylphenidate is comparable to 10 mg of methylphenidate in the morning and 10 mg in the early afternoon. Clinically, however, regular methylphenidate is superior for individual children in almost every case. We do not recommend the use of sustained-release methylphenidate.

Table 3.6

Dextroamphetamine Drug Interaction

Inhibits: • Beta-adrenergic blockers (propranolol)
In Combination with TCAs, MAOIs, Inhibiting Antidepressants, Narcotics: • Effects of both medications increased
Delays Absorption of: • Phenytoin • Phenobarbital • Ethosuximide
Decreases Hypotensive Effect of: • Guanethidine
Absorption Lowered by: • GI-acidifying agents
Absorption Increased by: • GI-alkalinizing agents
Renal Clearance Increased by: • Urine-acidifying agents
Renal Clearance Decreased by: • Urine-alkalinizing agents (i.e., thiazides)
Increases: • Plasma corticosteroid levels
May Alter: • Urinary steroid measurements • Insulin requirements

Dextroamphetamine

When methylphenidate is not effective, dextroamphetamine is the second line of treatment; 70 to 80% of children and adolescents will respond to this medication. Failure to respond

Table 3.7

Clinician's Guide to Using Stimulants for ADHD in Children and Adolescents

---

Methylphenidate Schedule:

- Not approved for children <6 years old
- Six years and older: Start with 5 mg twice a day, increase by 5–10 mg/week to maximum dose not to exceed 60 mg
- Optimal dose 0.3–0.7 mg/kg/dose two to three times per day (total daily dose: 0.9–2.1 mg/kg/day). Do not exceed 1 mg/kg/dose
- Therapeutic dose range 0.15–0.6 mg/kg/day
- Usual dose range 20–40 mg/day
- Extreme dose range 40–60 mg/day or higher

Dextroamphetamine Schedule:

- Not approved for children <3 years
- Three to five years: Start with 2.5 mg/day increased by 2.5 mg/week; adjust to best tolerated dose
- Six years and older: Start with 2.5 mg twice a day, increase by 5 mg/week to maximum dose not to exceed 40 mg
- Optimal dose 0.15–0.5 mg/kg two to three times daily (total daily dose: 0.3–1.5 mg/kg/day)
- Therapeutic dose range 0.08–0.3 mg/kg/day
- Usual dose range 10–20 mg/day
- Extreme dose range 30–40 mg/day

Pemoline Schedule:

- Not approved for children <6 years
- Six years and older: Start with 37.5 mg/day, increase by 18.75 mg/week to maximum daily dose of 112.5 mg/day
- Therapeutic dose range 0.6–4 mg/kg/day
- Usual dose range 37.5–112.5 mg/day
- Extreme dose range >112.5 mg/day

---

to methylphenidate does not predict similar failure or success of dextroamphetamine or magnesium pemoline.

Dextroamphetamine is safe, with few side effects, and with a short half-life slightly longer than that of methylphenidate (see Table 3.1). Growth suppression, anorexia, and weight loss are greater with dextroamphetamine than with methylphenidate, but rebound growth after the cessation of dextroamphetamine is greater.

Pemoline lacks sympathomimetic activity and is sometimes helpful when use of the other stimulants has resulted in problematic side effects. When other stimulants have precipitated a psychosis or severe tic disorder, pemoline should not be used.

Dextro and Levo Amphetamine (Adderall)

There is now a form of dextroamphetamine available which contains both dextro (d) and levo (l) amphetamine called Adderall. The advantage of this medication is that it appears that most patients can be treated on once or twice daily therapy (Data on File, Richwood Pharamecutical Company, Inc.). Of 611 children 3 to 12 years of age with ADHD studied, nearly 40% were able to be satisfactorily treated with once a day dosing and over 50% were able to be maintained on twice per day dosing. Only 7% of patients required dosing three or more times per day. The medication has a half-life of 8 to 12 hours. Its safety profile is similar to that of amphetamine products such as d-amphetamine. The most common side effects are those typical of d-amphetamine (see above) and include weight loss, decreased appetite, upset stomach, irritability and headache. Like other psychostimulants, when Adderall is used, the clinican must be on the alert for growth suppression, exacerbation or induction of tics and Tourette's syndrome and psychosis. Amphetamines such as Adderall do have significant potential for abuse, although when prescribed and taken correctly there have been no documented cases of addiction.

Dosing and Administration

The medication comes in 10 mg and 20 mg scored tablets. Starting doses of 2.5 mg per day are recommended for children 3 to 5 years of age. For children 6 years of age and older, medication can be started at 5 mg per day. The dose can then be increased by 2.5 mg per week in 3 to 5 year olds and by 5 mg per week in patients 6 years of age and older until maximal efficacy with minimal toxicity. Maximum recommended doses are 40 mg per day. Once daily dosing is often able to be achieved which may facilitate compliance. For added detail regarding the initiation and maintenance of treatment with this medication, please refer to the above section on dextroamphetamine.

Overdose

See Table 3.8.

Although an overdose with stimulants is less dangerous than overdosing with other medications, such as tricyclic antidepressants (TCAs) or lithium (see Chapters 4 and 8), careful monitoring is required when these medications are prescribed as children with ADHD have a higher suicide risk than do children without this disorder.

Table 3.8

Stimulant Overdose

Signs and Symptoms:
• Autonomic hyperactivity, i.e., hypertension, hyperthermia, and tachycardia • Psychosis • Cardiovascular complications • Seizure
Treatment:
• Close cardiac and respiratory monitoring • Chlorpromazine 50 mg PO/IM four times per day to treat paranoid psychosis since it is both antipsychotic and antihypertensive • Propranolol 1 mg IV every 5 minutes, with maximum dose of 8 mg for severe hypertension and tachycardia • Haloperidol 5 mg b.i.d. is better when hypertension is mild because it has fewer anticholinergic and sedating properties than chlorpromazine • If extra sedation is required because of psychosis, lorazepam 1–2 mg PO/IM is the best choice, as it is the only benzodiazepine with reliable IM absorption, and it is short-acting • Psychosis and delirium should clear within a few days if properly treated • If the patient is unconscious or having seizures, maintaining airway, breathing, circulation (ABCs) is critical • High fevers require medical management • Seizures can be treated with lorazepam or diazepam

Table 3.9

Signs and Symptoms of Stimulant Abuse When Taken in Large, Nontherapeutic Quantities

---

Acute Abuse:
- Sympathomimetic overload, i.e., hypertension, tachycardia, dry mouth, pupillary dilation
- Stereotyped behaviors
- Irritability and emotional lability
- Paranoia

Abuse

See Table 3.9.

Prescribing clinicians must be aware of the abuse potential of stimulants. Dextroamphetamine has the highest risk, methylphenidate has an intermediate risk, and pemoline has the lowest risk for abuse of all. Amphetamine abuse, both orally and IV, can have severe consequences, including necrotizing angiitis of the brain. Stimulants can produce a euphoric feeling initially that may be pleasing to pediatric patients with ADHD, who commonly suffer from low self-esteem. Persons taking methylphenidate and dextroamphetamine soon become tolerant to the euphorigenic and sympathomimetic effects, while tolerance is not seen in children and adolescents treated therapeutically with ADHD. Stimulant abusers tolerant to high doses of stimulants can tolerate doses that could kill or severely harm persons without tolerance. Psychological withdrawal after stimulant abuse is very common, but physical withdrawal does not occur. It is critical to monitor such patients closely during withdrawal as depressive symptoms with suicidal ideation are not uncommon.

References

1. Barkley, R.A. (1990). *Hyperactive Children: A Handbook for Diagnosis and Treatment*. New York: Guilford.
2. Pelham, W.E. (1989). Behavior therapy, behavioral assessment, and psychostimulant medication in the treatment of ADD: An interactive approach. In L. Bloomingdale, J. Swanson, R. Klorman

(Eds.), *Attention Deficit Disorders: New Directions* (vol. 4) (pp. 169–195). New York: Spectrum.

3. Lucas, A.R., Weiss, M. (1971). Methylphenidate hallucinosis. *JAMA, 217*, 1079–1081.

4. Barkley, R.A., Anastopoulos, D.C., Guevremont, D.C. (1991). Adolescents with ADHD: Patterns of behavioral adjustment, academic functioning, and treatment utilization. *J Am Acad Child Adolesc Psychiatry, 30*, 752–761.

5. Wender, P. (1987). *The Hyperactive Child, Adolescent, and Adult: Attention Deficit Disorder Through the Lifespan.* New York: Oxford University Press.

6. Kaplan, H.I., Sadock, B.J. (1991). *Synopsis of Psychiatry* (6th ed.) (pp. 658–660). Baltimore: Williams & Wilkins.

7. *Physicians' Desk Reference* (50th ed.) (1996). Oradell, N.J.: Medical Economics.

8. Forrest, W.H., Brown, B., Brown, C.R., et al. (1977). Dextroamphetamine with morphine for the treatment of postoperative pain. *N Engl J Med, 296*, 712.

9. Safer, D.J., Allen, R.P., Barr, E. (1972). Depression in growth in hyperactive children on stimulant drugs. *N Engl J Med, 287*, 217–220.

10. Safer, D.J., Allen, R.P. (1973). Factors influencing the suppressant effects of two stimulant drugs on the growth of hyperactive children. *Pediatrics, 51*, 660–667.

Tricyclic Antidepressants

The antidepressant drugs are a heterogenous group of compounds that, in adults, have been found to be effective in the treatment of major depressive disorder, generalized anxiety disorder, panic disorder, and a variety of other conditions. In this section, we focus on the tricyclic antidepressants (TCAs). Antidepressants of other classes, such as fluoxetine, sertraline, paroxetine, fluvoxamine, venlafaxine, bupropion, trazodone, and nefazadone, are discussed in Chapter 5.

The TCAs have long been the first-line antidepressants used by most clinicians for adults because of their established efficacy, safety, and ease of administration, but they have been less successful in the treatment of child and adolescent conditions. This is particularly true of childhood and adolescent depression, where there is no conclusive evidence that TCAs are superior to placebo. Nonetheless, investigation has revealed other potential roles for TCAs in the treatment of childhood and adolescent psychiatric conditions.

Chemical Properties

The mechanism by which TCAs are effective in the treatment of adult depression and other disorders has not been clearly established. There is, however, evidence that these agents affect monoamine neurotransmitter systems in the central nervous system (CNS), such as serotonin and norepinephrine.[1] The TCAs block the reuptake of norepinephrine and serotonin, potentiating their action. It has been suggested that antidepressants work by increasing noradrenergic and/or serotonergic transmission, compensating for a presumed deficiency.

Indications

See Table 4.1.

Major Depressive Disorder

Controlled studies have failed to demonstrate that TCAs are superior to placebo in the treatment of childhood and adolescent depression.[2–7] Clinicians continue to prescribe these agents, however, in the belief that future studies will show that higher plasma levels or correctly adjusted doses of antidepressants will be effective. There are data that strongly indicate continuity from child and adolescent depression to adult forms of the disorder. There also seem to be similarities in psychobiological correlates.

Current Practice

As mentioned above, despite the fact that TCAs have not been proved effective in the treatment of major depressive disorder (MDD), their use for children and adolescents is widespread, and is even considered standard practice in many clinical settings. A child with a family member who has responded well to a particular TCA may merit a trial of the same agent. As in adults with MDD, antidepressant treatment is typically maintained for 9 to 12 months before a gradual tapering off is initiated. In adults, maintenance therapy at doses comparable to those used

Table 4.1

Tricyclic Antidepressants:
Clinical Indications

Established Indications:
- Enuresis
- ADHD in children and adolescents

Probable Indications:
- ADHD in adults
- School absenteeism/school phobia
- OCD (serotonergic agents only)
- Depression

to treat peak depressive symptoms can reduce the risk of relapse of a depressive episode. This option may be considered in children or adolescents who have not experienced any undue side effects. We suggest discussing these options with the child and parents before recommending a specific treatment course.

Attention-Deficit Hyperactivity Disorder

Up to 30% of children treated with stimulants for ADHD do not improve, necessitating alternative treatments.[8,9] Imipramine, desipramine, and amitriptyline have been shown to be superior to placebo in treating ADHD.[10] However, most studies find stimulants to be superior to antidepressants.

Coexisting Tics

The existence of tic symptoms may warrant a TCA trial. These agents have the advantage that they are effective in the treatment of ADHD, but do not exacerbate tics as stimulants can. We recommend using desipramine as the first antidepressant in the treatment of ADHD and tics. This antidepressant has a relatively favorable side-effect profile. It should be noted that desipramine is not an effective treatment of tic disorders.

Enuresis

Enuresis remains the only Food and Drug Administration (FDA)–established indication for the use of TCAs in children. Desipramine and imipramine, which are equally efficacious, are the only antidepressants approved for the treatment of enuresis. Imipramine has more side effects, but is less expensive. It is recommended that desipramine be reserved for patients who have both diurnal and nocturnal enuresis, and for those whose nocturnal enuresis has not responded to conservative behavioral measures. Clomipramine has also been used to treat enuresis, with a therapeutic effect observed at plasma concentrations of 20 to 60 ng/ml. Pharmacologic approaches should not be employed until all organic etiologies are ruled out by physical and laboratory examination.

1-Deamino-8-d-Arginine-Vasopressin (DDAVP)

Pediatricians often use DDAVP as the medication treatment of first choice in enuretic children, while using TCAs less frequently.

Anxiety/Panic/Phobic Disorders

There are very limited data on the treatment of panic disorder, phobic disorder, and anxiety disorder in children and adolescents. Although TCAs are used, we advise initiating treatment using a low dose of a selective serotonin reuptake inhibitor (SSRI) (see Chapter 5). Despite the lack of controlled studies of SSRIs for these conditions in children and adolescents, clinicians frequently implement low-dose SSRI treatment because of the favorable side-effect profile.

Obsessive-Compulsive Disorder

Clomipramine is an antiobsessional drug that has been found to be effective in the treatment of adult and pediatric obsessive-compulsive disorder (OCD).

Contraindications

See Table 4.2.

A history of hypersensitivity to TCAs is a contraindication to TCA therapy. A TCA should not be administered while a patient is receiving an MAOI, and should not be initiated until the patient has been off the MAOI for at least two weeks. An MAOI can be added to an ongoing TCA regimen that has only been partially effective. Adding an MAOI to a TCA is relatively safe for desipramine and nortriptyline, but is contraindicated when

Table 4.2

Contraindications to TCA Therapy

Absolute:
• Prior hypersensitivity reaction
• Currently on MAOI
Relative:
• Pregnancy
• Epilepsy
• Psychosis (i.e., schizophrenia)
• Cardiac problem
• Thyroid condition

imipramine or amitriptyline is being administered. Imipramine is even more toxic than amitriptyline when used in combination with MAOIs. In general, TCAs should be avoided during pregnancy. Since TCAs are secreted in breast milk, mothers should be discouraged from breast-feeding if they are taking TCAs. TCAs can lower the seizure threshold. When a patient is on a stable anticonvulsant regimen, this is generally not problematic. As TCAs can induce or exacerbate psychosis, we do not advocate their use for psychotic children and adolescents. Cardiac disorders must be approached cautiously when TCA therapy is considered (see "Side Effects"). The use of TCAs in patients with thyroid dysfunction also must be approached cautiously, because this condition can induce arrhythmias.

Side Effects

See Table 4.3.

Mild increases in PR and QRS intervals are common in children and adolescents treated with TCAs. A mild increase in the pulse rate of up to 120 beats per minute is not uncommon, and is

Table 4.3

Side Effects of TCAs in Children and Adolescents

- Anticholinergic
- Anxiety
- Cardiac
- Confusion
- Hypertension
- Incoordination
- Insomnia/nightmares
- Mania
- Photosensitization
- Psychosis
- Rash
- Seizures
- Sexual dysfunction
- Tics
- Tremor

frequently asymptomatic. Greater cardiac conduction slowing (i.e., PR > 0.21 and QRS > 0.12) can be dangerous, and can result in arrhythmias and/or heart block. Of greatest concern are the reports of sudden cardiac deaths of children on TCAs; three cases involved desipramine and one involved imipramine. These sudden deaths have generated concern regarding the safety of TCAs for young children, especially at doses greater than 3.5 mg/kg. Treatment with TCAs at doses above 3.5 mg/kg or at plasma levels greater than 150 ng/ml may increase the risk of asymptomatic ECG changes, particularly a slight prolongation of the PR interval and moderate increases in the QRS duration. Delayed cardiac conduction and minor increases in diastolic blood pressure and heart rate can also be seen. At the present time, no causal link between sudden cardiac death and TCA use has been established. Nonetheless, the potential risk and other side effects need to be taken into account when TCA therapy is considered. Although clinicians should not be so alarmed that they refuse to prescribe such medications, careful monitoring is essential in these patients. See Table 4.4 for ECG and blood pressure guidelines for the use of TCAs.

Anticholinergic side effects, such as dry mouth and constipation, are frequent side effects in children and adolescents, but are usually not dose-limiting and often dissipate with time. Blurred vision and urinary retention occur much less commonly in children and adolescents than in adults. Psychosis and mania are uncommon but potentially serious side effects of TCA therapy. All of the antidepressants can decrease the seizure threshold, although this side effect is uncommon. The risk of seizures is highest in children and adolescents with neurologic disorders, abnormal electroencephalograms (EEGs), and/or abnormal neurologic examination. Maprotiline is the TCA most associated with increasing the risk of seizures, leading many investigators to call for its withdrawal. Hypertension is an uncommon side effect and is usually clinically significant only when there is preexisting hypertension. Confusion most often is secondary to anticholinergic toxicity, and has been reported with higher TCA plasma levels. An allergic reaction to TCA therapy is relatively rare. Tics, tremor, and incoordination are occasional side effects of TCAs. Breast enlargement and galactorrhea have been reported occasionally in females treated

Table 4.4

ECG and Blood Pressure Guidelines for the Use of TCAs for Children and Adolescents

---

A. ECG

Baseline ECG must be done in all patients before starting treatment with TCAs (for ECG, blood pressure, and pulse parameters, see below).

For doses greater than 25 mg/day, ECG rhythm strip should be obtained before each TCA dose increase or when the TCA reaches the steady state (three to five days).

During maintenance, ECGs or rhythm strips will be repeated at least once every three months. TCAs will be reduced or discontinued if:

PR interval: Patient $\leq$10 years of age and PR interval is >0.18. Patient is >10 years old and PR interval is >0.20.

QRS interval: >0.12 second or widening more than 50% over baseline QRS interval.

Corrected QT: $\geq$0.48 second.

Heart rate: Patient is $\leq$10 years of age and *resting supine* heart rate is >110. Patient is >10 years of age and *resting supine* rate is >100.

B. Blood Pressure (BP)*

The child should be in a comfortable sitting or supine position and *sufficient time should be allowed for recovery from recent activity or apprehension.*

For inpatients, blood pressure and pulse should be measured at least three times a week.

For outpatients, during dose titration, blood pressure and pulse should be taken at least once a week.

During maintenance, blood pressure and pulse should be taken at least once a month (if it is possible, we recommend that the school nurse take more frequent blood pressure and pulse readings and call us if the patient has questionable readings or they meet the criteria for lowering or discontinuing TCAs).

The manometer must be well calibrated and proper cuff size should be used (long enough to completely encircle the circumference of the arm—with or without overlap—and wide enough to cover approximately 75% of the upper arm between the top of the shoulder and the olecranon).

TCAs will be reduced or discontinued if:

(Continued)

Table 4.4

(Continued)

Patient is ≤10 years of age and *resting* BP ≥ 140/90 or if BP is persistently greater than 130/85 (50% of the time during three weeks).
Patient is >10 years of age and *resting* BP ≥ 150/95 or persistently greater than 140/85 (50% of the time during three weeks).

C. Patients who must continue treatment with TCAs and have questionable or borderline BP and/or ECG or meet the above criteria for lowering or discontinuing TCAs will be referred to the pediatric cardiology department at Children's Hospital for further evaluation and Holter monitoring.

D. Lying and standing blood pressure and pulse may be obtained to assess possible orthostatic hypotension at the discretion of the physician.

Note: These criteria were developed by Dr. James Zuberbuhler (Chief, Department of Pediatric Cardiology) and Dr. Lee Beerman, both from Children's Hospital of Pittsburgh. The guidelines are empirical and subject to change.
*The BP guidelines were made under the assumption that patients will remain on treatment with TCAs for six to nine months.

with TCAs, and gynecomastia has been seen in males. Increased and decreased libido and impotence have also been observed.

Drug Interactions

See Table 4.5.

Clinical Practice

For the dosing and administration of specific agents, see Tables 4.6 through 4.9.

Prior to initiating a TCA trial, children and adolescents should have a physical examination, including the measurement of heart rate, blood pressure, weight, and height. A baseline ECG is required, and thereafter, ECG rhythm strip, blood pressure, and pulse should be obtained at each dose increase and at frequent intervals during dose elevation. A pregnancy test and evaluation for adequate contraceptive use are advised in females of child-bearing age. Patients should be observed for tics and involuntary movements on starting medication.

Table 4.5

Drug Interactions of TCAs

May Increase Effect of:
• Alcohol
• Anticholinergic agents
• Antipsychotics
• Barbiturates
• Benzodiazepines
• CNS stimulants
• CNS depressants
• MAOIs
• Phenytoin
• Seizure-potentiating drugs
• Sympathomimetics (i.e., ephedrine)
• Thyroid medications (cardiac effects)
May Decrease Effect of:
• Clonidine
• Guanethidine
Effects may be Increased by:
• Marijuana (tachycardia)
• Methylphenidate
• Oral contraceptives (estrogen)
• Phenothiazines

Table 4.6

Dosage and Regimen of TCAs in Major Depressive Disorder

Imipramine and Desipramine:
• Used at doses up to 5.0 mg/kg/day
• Start with dose 75 mg/day
• After 7–10 days, draw serum desipramine and imipramine levels
• Children and adolescents treated with serum levels effective in adult MDD
• Usually increased to achieve serum levels >150 ng/ml as in adults
• Serum levels >150 ng/ml may increase risk for ECG abnormalities (i.e., increased heart rate, conduction abnormalities)(may be of more statistical than clinical significance)
• Careful monitoring required

Table 4.7

Dosage and Regimen of TCAs for ADHD

Desipramine and Imipramine: • Optimal doses 2.5–5 mg/kg/day • Should not exceed serum levels >300 ng/ml • No significant correlation between serum level, dosage, and clinical response • Serum levels >150 ng/ml and doses >3.5 mg/kg/day associated with increased risk of heart rate and altered cardiac conduction • ECG PR <200 ms and QRS <120 ms advocated • Daily doses >5 mg/kg/day may be needed clinically to achieve serum levels >150 ng/ml • Doses >3.5 mg/kg may be too much for some children • Careful monitoring required
Nortriptyline: • Has not been systematically studied • May be considered if imipramine or desipramine is unsuccessful or contraindicated • Careful monitoring required
Amitriptyline, Clomipramine, Doxepin, and Maprotiline: • Not recommended for use

Plasma antidepressant levels should be drawn five to seven days after the last dose increase, and 12 hours after the most recently administered dose. Children and adolescents should have an annual physical examination by their pediatrician or family practitioner. Dry mouth is a frequently encountered side effect and may be ameliorated by reducing the dose, or by using sugar-free gum or candy.

As these agents have a potential for causing death, either in accidental or deliberate overdose (see "Overdose"), they must be kept under careful supervision. Locking them away in child-protective containers is advised. We advocate prescribing no more than a two-week supply of medication at one time.

There are no firm guidelines as to treatment duration with TCAs for children and adolescents with psychiatric disorders. Our recommendations (see "Clinical Indications") are based on a

Table 4.8

Dosage and Regimen of TCAs for Enuresis

Desipramine:
- Typical doses 1–2.5 mg/kg/day
- Doses of 50–75 mg/day usually sufficient
- Antienuretic effects occur soon after treatment initiated
- Antienuretic effect not related to anticholinergic mechanism
- Relationship of serum level to clinical outcome not clear
- Routine clinical practice: ECGs not usually done as final daily dose is usually ≤2.5 mg/kg/day
- Risk of cardiotoxicity low at these doses
- *We recommend baseline ECGs and serial ECG rhythm strips after each dose increase, owing to recent reports of sudden cardiac death*

Clomipramine:
- Effective
- Targeted plasma concentrations: 20–60 ng/ml
- Plasma levels <20 ng/ml and >60 ng/ml associated with lack of efficacy
- Use only if desipramine and imipramine ineffective

Amitriptyline, Doxepin, Maprotiline, and Nortriptyline:
- Not recommended for use

Table 4.9

Dosage and Regimen of TCAs in Childhood and Adolescent OCD

Clomipramine:
- TCA of choice
- Superior to other antidepressants
- Side effects can be problematic
- Initial dose: 25 mg/day for children <25 kg, 50 mg/day if >25 kg
- Increase dosage weekly by amount equal to subject's initial dose
- Maximum daily dose should not exceed 5 mg/kg or 250 mg
- Combination therapy may exacerbate problematic fluoxetine side effects (i.e., akathisia)
- Careful monitoring required

Other TCAs not recommended

---

review of the available literature and on clinical experience. Children are at higher risk than adults for experiencing withdrawal symptoms when TCAs are discontinued. They commonly show daily withdrawal effects on regular once-a-day dosing. Therefore, the agents often need to be given in two or three divided doses daily for children and adolescents. Withdrawal symptoms from TCAs include anxiety, agitation, disrupted sleep, behavioral activation, and flulike symptoms, such as somatic or GI distress. These side effects can be minimized or avoided by gradually tapering the medication over two weeks. Finally, we recommend SSRIs as first-line agents in the treatment of pediatric depression given their more favorable side-effect profile and preliminary evidence that SSRIs (fluoxetine) are superior to placebo in treating this illness (see Chapter 5).

Overdose

See Table 4.10.

Table 4.10

TCA Overdose

Signs and Symptoms:
- Antimuscarinic effects, i.e., dry mucous membranes, warm dry skin, blurred vision, and mydriasis
- Heart arrhythmias and cardiac arrest
- Respiratory arrest
- Seizures
- Hypotension
- Drowsiness/coma
- High potential for causing death, especially if more than 1 gram is ingested
- Symptoms develop within 24 hours of overdose
- Plasma antidepressant levels may not reflect severity of overdose
- Side effects exacerbated if other CNS depressants are ingested

Treatment of Overdose:
- Close cardiac and respiratory monitoring

(Continued)

Table 4.10

(*Continued*)

- Epinephrine for hypotension to counteract anti–alpha-adrenergic side effects of TCA
- Continuous cardiac monitoring in ICU for any patient with arrhythmias and/or QRS greater than 0.12
- Monitor serum TCA levels and cardiac function until arrhythmias and QRS have normalized and plasma antidepressants are no longer toxic.
- Sinus tachycardia often does *not* necessitate treatment
- Direct-current cardioversion may be indicated for supraventricular tachycardia causing hypotension or myocardial ischemia
- Propranolol is safe and effective in the treatment of recurrent supraventricular tachycardia
- Digoxin *contraindicated*, can precipitate heart block
- Cardioversion is treatment of choice for ventricular tachycardia or ventricular fibrillation
- Administration of loading dose of lidocaine and a drip of 2 mg/min may decrease risk recurrence
- If lidocaine is unsuccessful in alleviating arrhythmias, propranolol and bretylium are indicated
- Quinidine, disopyramide, and procainamide are *contraindicated* for TCA overdose—may prolong QRS and precipitate heart block
- Physostigmine is *not* effective in treating TCA-induced arrhythmias
- Temporary pacemakers may be necessary for second- and third-degree heart block
- If alert, emesis induction is indicated
- Intubation and gastric lavage if not alert
- Administer 30 grams of activated charcoal with 120 cc of magnesium citrate to reduce absorption of residual drug, since bowel mobility may have been slowed
- For seizures, administer diazepam 5–10 mg IV at rate of 2 mg/min; may repeat every 5–10 minutes until seizures are controlled
- Minimize risk of respiratory decompensation by administering IV benzodiapazines slowly
- Lorazepam may have lower risk of respiratory decompensation; administer 1–2 mg IV over several minutes. Also has longer effect when administered acutely (hours vs. minutes)
- If benzodiapazines are unsuccessful, phenytoin is indicated. Give loading dose of 15 mg/kg, not exceeding 50 mg/min
- Forced diuresis and dialyses are not helpful and may increase hemodynamic compromise

The TCAs have a very high potential for causing death when taken in overdose, even if the child is brought to the hospital immediately after the event. When a patient overdoses on more than 1 gram of a TCA, toxicity often results and death can occur.

Abuse

The TCAs have a very low risk for abuse.

References

1. Arana, G.W., Hyman, S.E. (Eds.) (1991). *Handbook of Psychiatric Drug Therapy* (2nd ed.) (pp. 38–78). Boston: Little Brown.
2. Puig-Antich, J., Perel, J.M., Lupatkin, W., et al. (1987). Imipramine in prepubertal major depressive disorders. *Arch Gen Psychiatry*, *44*, 81–89.
3. Geller, B., Cooper, T.B., McCombs, H.G., et al. (1989). Double-blind, placebo-controlled study of nortriptyline in depressed children using a "fixed plasma level" design. *Psychopharmacol Bull*, *25*, 101–108.
4. Kramer, A.D., Feiguine, R.J. (1981). Clinical effects of amitriptyline in adolescent depression: A pilot study. *J Am Acad Child Psychiatry*, *20*, 636–644.
5. Geller, B., et al. (1989). A double-blind, placebo-controlled study of nortriptyline in adolescents with major depression (abstract). Washington, DC: National Institute of Mental Health New Clinical Drug Evaluation Unit (NCDEU) Annual Meeting.
6. Ryan, N.D., Puig-Antich, J., Cooper, T.B., et al. (1986). Imipramine in adolescent major depression: Plasma level and clinical response. *Acta Psychiatr Scand*, *73*, 275–288.
7. Strober, M. (1989). Effects of imipramine, lithium, and fluoxetine in the treatment of adolescent major depression (abstract). Washington, DC: National Institute of Mental Health New Clinical Drug Evaluation Unit (NCDEU) Annual Meeting.
8. Rapoport, J.L., Zametkin, A. (1980). ADD. *Psychiatr Clin N Am*, *3*, 425–442.
9. Barkley, R.A. (1977). A review of stimulant drug research with hyperactive children. *J Child Psychol Psychiatry*, *18*, 137–165.
10. Garfinkel, B.D., Wender, P.H., Sloman, L., et al. (1983). Tricyclic antidepressants and methylphenidate treatment of ADD in children. *J Am Acad Child Psychiatry*, *22*, 343–348.

C h a p t e r 5

SSRIs and
Newer Antidepressants

The selective serotonin reuptake inhibitors (SSRIs), fluoxetine, fluvoxamine, paroxetine, and sertraline, have become popular, and are often the drugs of first choice, because of their lack of anticholinergic and cardiac side effects. Bupropion, trazodone, nefazodone, and venlafaxine, antidepressants that are not chemically related to the TCAs or the SSRIs, are approved for treating depression in adults.

Fluoxetine

Fluoxetine has no direct effect on other neurotransmitter systems or receptor sites.[1] Thus, it and other members of its class are relatively safe in overdose. The starting and maintenance dose in adults is 20 mg/day. Efficacy and safety have not yet been clearly established for children and adolescents, but its clinical use in this population has been increasing.

Fluoxetine is metabolized primarily by the liver. Active and inactive metabolites are excreted in the urine by the kidneys. At standard doses of 20 mg/day in adults, fluoxetine achieves peak plasma levels after six to eight hours. However, a 10-mg starting dose may be more appropriate in children. Its primary active metabolite, norfluoxetine, has a half-life of seven to nine days. Fluoxetine is highly protein bound (95%).

Emslie et al. (1997) have completed an important clinical trial of fluoxetine in adolescent outpatients (7 to 17 years) with

DSM-III-R criteria for non-psychotic major depressive disorder (MDD). The dosage used was fluoxetine 20 mg or placebo and they were seen weekly for eight consecutive weeks. The study demonstrated that of the 96 subjects, 48 were randomized to fluoxetine and 48 to placebo. Using the intent-to-treat sample, 27 (56%) of those on fluoxetine and 16 (33%) on placebo were rated much or very much improved on the CGI at study termination. $P \leq 0.024$.

Significant differences were also noted in other weekly ratings after five weeks of treatment, but it is important to note that complete symptom remission (CDRS-R $\leq$ 28) occurs in only 31% of fluoxetine treated and 23% of placebo treated subjects.[2]

Sertraline

Sertraline has a much shorter half-life and fewer side effects than fluoxetine. Sertraline does not increase plasma levels of other psychotropic medications to the same extent as does fluoxetine.[3] Its efficacy has also been demonstrated in MDD and OCD in adults, but has not been established in children.[4-6] In adults the treatment is initiated with a dose of 50 mg once daily. While a relationship between dose and antidepressant effect has not been established, patients were dosed in a range of 50–200 mg/day in the clinical trials. The average terminal elimination half-life of plasma sertraline is about 26 hours.

Paroxetine

Paroxetine, like sertraline, has a much shorter half-life and fewer side effects than fluoxetine. The recommended initial dose is 20 mg/day in adults. Patients were dosed in a range of 20–50 mg/day in the clinical trials. The half-life of paroxetine is approximately 20 hours (see Table 5.1).

Paroxetine is well-absorbed from the GI tract and is extracted as pharmacologically inactive metabolites. Steady-state plasma concentration occurs within 7–14 days. With this agent as with the other SSRI's there appears to be no association between plasma concentrations and efficacy or side effects in adults.

All the SSRIs are chemically unrelated to the TCAs. They do not affect norepinephrine or dopamine uptake.

Table 5.1

Comparison of Clinical Profiles of SSRIs

	Fluoxetine	Fluvoxamine	Paroxetine	Sertraline
Half-life	24–72 hrs	15 hrs	20 hrs	25 hrs
Increases plasma levels of other psychotropic medications	More	Less	Less	Less
Overall side effects	More	Less	Less	Less
Increased anxiety and restlessness	More	Less	Less	Less

In contrast to fluoxetine, the principal metabolites of the others have been shown to be significantly less active than the parent compounds. Sertraline and paroxetine, like fluoxetine, are highly protein bound (95–98%), and fluvoxamine is slightly less so at 77%.

Indications

See Table 5.2.

Major Depressive Disorder

In adults, placebo-controlled studies have shown the SSRIs' therapeutic effectiveness in outpatients to be similar to that of the TCAs.[7] One placebo-controlled study reports fluoxetine's effectiveness in the treatment of childhood and adolescent depression.[8]

Children and adolescents may require a lower starting dose of 5 to 10 mg/day of fluoxetine for the first week, which should be

Table 5.2

Indications for SSRIs in Child and Adolescent Psychiatry

FDA-Established Indications:
- None

Probable Indications:
- MDD/dysthymia
- OCD

Possible Indications:
- ADHD
- Trichotillomania
- Compulsive impulse control disorders
- Panic disorder
- Anorexia nervosa
- Bulimia nervosa
- Prader-Willi syndrome
- Self-injurious behavior
- Borderline personality disorder
- Posttraumatic stress syndrome
- Drug craving

increased only if improvement is not evident. A trial of six to eight weeks may be required before resistance to fluoxetine is inferred.

Fluoxetine may also be useful in treating OCD (see Table 5.2).[9] Higher doses are usually required than for depression. Fluoxetine-clomipramine combinations have been utilized to maximize therapeutic response and minimize toxicity with some limited success.[10] Very limited data are available, and further study is necessary before this strategy can be endorsed. Fluvoxamine and sertraline[11] have also been found to be effective in the treatment of adult OCD. There are no published controlled studies establishing paroxetine's efficacy in OCD. There are no data on children or adolescents.

Trichotillomania and Other Compulsive-Impulsive Control Disorders

The serotonergic agent clomipramine has been found effective in the treatment of trichotillomania (a disorder believed to have an OCD component) and in the treatment of autistic children with disturbances in social relatedness, obsessive-compulsive symptoms, impulse control problems, and/or aggressive behaviors[12] (see "Indications", Chapter 4). Although there are no data on fluoxetine, it makes sense that this agent may be helpful for some of these patients.

Attention-Deficit Hyperactivity Disorder

Fluoxetine has been tried in an open trial of ADHD with a positive report of efficacy. The children and adolescents in this study received 20 to 60 mg/day. To date, there have been no controlled studies demonstrating fluoxetine's efficacy in this condition. There are no data on the other SSRIs and other newer atypical agents in the treatment of ADHD.

Bulimia Nervosa

The SSRIs may be the ideal agents for this disorder.[13-17] The cycle of binging and purging in bulimia has often been characterized as having a compulsive and/or obsessive quality, for which the SSRIs may be especially effective. Bulimic patients are notoriously prone to impulsive acts, such as suicide attempts. The SSRIs are less lethal in overdose than are the TCAs (see "Overdose/Toxicity" on p. 49).

Table 5.3

Contraindications to Using SSRIs

- Known hypersensitivity reaction
- On MAOI within past five weeks (fluoxetine) or past two weeks (sertraline)
- Pregnancy
- Liver disease
- On terfenadine (Seldane)

See Table 5.3.

Patients on MAOIs

Fluoxetine and sertraline should not be prescribed to any patient who has received an MAOI within two weeks. Conversely, an MAOI should not be started within five weeks of using fluoxetine (see Chapter 6). In patients receiving both fluoxetine and an MAOI, there have been reports of severe, sometimes fatal, reactions. Some cases had features resembling those of the neuroleptic malignant syndrome.

Pregnancy

These medications can cross the placenta and should be avoided by nursing mothers.

Side Effects

See Table 5.4.

Gastrointestinal Complaints

Gastrointestinal complaints, such as nausea, diarrhea, and dyspepsia, are common side effects in patients treated with SSRIs. Weight loss and decreased appetite are fairly common side effects with fluoxetine.

Nervousness and Insomnia

Nervousness, insomnia, and tense feelings are common side effects of SSRIs. In adults, trazodone, 25 to 50 mg at bedtime, has proved helpful for fluoxetine-induced insomnia.[18] In a patient suffering from insomnia, the clinician should be alert for possibly evolving hypomania/mania, particularly if other manic-like symptoms become evident.

Table 5.4

Side Effects of Fluoxetine, Sertraline, Paroxetine, and Fluvoxamine

Common:
- GI (nausea, vomiting, diarrhea, dyspepsia)
- Decreased appetite
- Weight loss (fluoxetine only)
- Nervousness, agitation, tremor, akathisia
- Insomnia
- Excess sweating
- Sedation
- Dream intensification (fluoxetine > sertraline, paroxetine, and fluvoxamine)
- Motor restlessness
- Dry mouth
- Male sexual dysfunction, anorgasmia

Occasional:
- Social disinhibition
- Subjective sensation of excitation
- Hypomania/mania
- Rash/allergic reactions
- Seizure
- Hair loss

Side Effects of Heterocyclic Agents Not Seen:
- Anticholinergic
- Cardiovascular

Note: There is no evidence that self-destructive phenomena (i.e., suicidal ideation/attempts) are more common with fluoxetine than with other antidepressants.

Dreaming
Abnormal dreams are a frequent side effect.

Motor Restlessness/Akathisia
Riddle and colleagues[19] observed motor restlessness, a relatively common side effect of SSRIs, in 46% of children and

adolescents treated with fluoxetine, 20 to 40 mg/day, for depressive or obsessive-compulsive symptoms.[20] Three children with ADHD actually showed an exacerbation of symptoms while on fluoxetine.

Neuromuscular restlessness can approximate neuroleptic-induced akathisia, and may respond to a dosage reduction or temporary benzodiazepine therapy.[18] Clonazepam, 0.25 to 0.5 mg b.i.d., has proved useful in treating this akathisia-like syndrome.[18]

Male Sexual Dysfunction

In adults, male sexual dysfunction, primarily ejaculatory delay, is considered to be a relatively common side affect of sertraline. Anorgasmia has been reported to affect approximately 5% of patients treated with fluoxetine.[21] This side effect may respond to cyproheptadine taken orally four to eight hours before sexual activity is planned.[22] There are no data on children and adolescents, although it is believed that the side effect is less common in this population.

Mania/Hypomania

Various reports describing mania induced by fluoxetine have surfaced.[23-25]

Seizures

Events described as seizures have been reported at a rate of 0.6%, a rate comparable to that observed with other antidepressants.[26] There are no data on the other SSRIs, but similar precautions are recommended.

Overdose/Toxicity

In contrast to the TCAs, overdoses with SSRIs have a low lethality. Symptoms of fluoxetine overdose can include agitation, nervousness, restlessness, nausea, vomiting, insomnia, seizures, hypomania/mania, and other signs of CNS excitation.[26]

The management of fluoxetine overdose involves establishing and maintaining an airway to ensure adequate oxygenation and ventilation.[26] Activated charcoal with sorbitol may be more effective than emesis or lavage. It is important that cardiac and

Table 5.5

Drug Interactions with SSRIs*

Coadministration can Result in Dangerous Side Effects for Patients on:
• MAOIs • Heterocyclics • L-tryptophan • Lithium • Seldane
When Used with These Agents, Increases Plasma Levels of:
• Heterocyclic antidepressants • Benzodiazepines (i.e., diazepam)
Coadministration can Result in Decreased Therapeutic Effect of:
• Buspirone
*Side effects of SSRIs likely are similar, although, in some cases, may be less severe or prolonged due to their shorter half-life.

vital signs be monitored during the acute period of the overdose. In addition to questioning the patient and family, urine and serum drug screens must be performed to adequately gauge what substances the patient ingested.

Drug Interactions

See Table 5.5.

Withdrawal

Intolerance to one SSRI does not mean that the patient will be intolerant to all others. In fact, recent findings in adults suggest that this does not happen.

See Table 5.6.

Clinical Practice

Dosing and Administration

For the use of benzodiazepines, see Chapter 10. Also see Tables 5.7 through 5.10.

Table 5.6

Parent Information on Fluoxetine

What is Prozac?

Prozac (generic name fluoxetine) is a medication that was developed as an antidepressant. It is chemically different from other antidepressant medications, and works in a different way. It is available in capsules (called Pulvules) and in a liquid form.

How can This Medication Help?

Because Prozac is so new, there has not been much research on its use with children and adolescents, although a great deal is known about its use with adults. It is being used on a trial basis to help children and adolescents who suffer from depression, OCD, or obsessions or compulsions as part of Tourette's syndrome. It may be effective for patients who have tried other medications, but do not get better or develop side effects.

How will the Doctor Monitor This Medicine?

The doctor will want you to have regular visits to evaluate how Prozac is working, to adjust the dose, to watch for side effects, and to see if other treatment is needed.

What Side Effects can This Medicine Have?

Any medication may have side effects. Because each patient is different, your doctor will work with you to get the most positive effects and the fewest negative effects from the medicine. This list may not include rare or unusual side effects. Please talk to the doctor if you suspect that the medicine is causing a problem. In general, Prozac has fewer and less troublesome side effects than other antidepressants.

Common Nuisance Side Effects:

Nausea, weight loss or gain, anxiety or nervousness, insomnia (trouble sleeping), excessive sweating, headaches.

Some persons may become restless or agitated, with increased activity and rapid speech and an uncomfortable feeling of being "speeded up." This is worse at first, and may improve if the dose is lowered.

There has been a lot of publicity suggesting that Prozac may cause suicidal thoughts. This is very rare, if it occurs at all, and may be due to the depression itself rather than to Prozac. In any case, if suicidal thoughts or actions appear or worsen, call the doctor right away.

(Continued)

Table 5.6

(Continued)

What Else Should I Know about This Medicine?

It can be dangerous to take Prozac at the same time or within five to six
weeks of taking a type of antidepressant called an MAO inhibitor (Nardil,
Parnate, or Marplan).

Prozac interacts with many other medications. Be sure each doctor knows all
of the medications that are being taken, or have been taken in the past
several months.

Source: Dulcan, M.K. (1992). Information for parents and youth on
psychotropic medications. *J Child Adolesc Psychopharmacol, 2,* 81–101.

Table 5.7

**Dosage and Administration of Fluoxetine, Sertraline,
Paroxetine, and Fluvoxamine in Child and Adolescent MDD**

Fluoxetine:
- Not proved effective by controlled study
- Open-label studies indicate possible efficacy
- To minimize side effects, low-dose therapy is recommended
- Therapeutic response may be seen at doses as low as 5 mg/day
- Initiate dose at 5 mg/day and increase by 5 mg every 7 to 10 days to
  maximum dose of 20 mg/day
- Lowest effective dose should be prescribed
- Medication trial of six to eight weeks necessary before treatment
  resistance can be determined
- Once treatment response occurs, must be maintained on medication
  for 9 to 12 months
- Still experimental
- Careful monitoring required

Sertraline:
- Not proved effective by controlled study
- No open-label studies
- Doses over 100 mg should be given b.i.d.
- Six- to eight-week trial is necessary before treatment resistance can be
  determined
- If treatment response occurs, maintain on medication 9 to 12 months
- Consider maintenance medication therapy

(Continued)

Table 5.7

(*Continued*)

- Experimental
- Careful monitoring required

Paroxetine:
- Not proved effective by controlled study
- No open-label studies
- Initial dose at 10 mg/day and increase by 10 mg every seven days to maximum dose of 50 mg/day
- Six- to eight-week trial is necessary before treatment resistance can be determined
- If treatment response occurs, maintain on medication 9 to 12 months
- Consider maintenance medication therapy
- Experimental
- Careful monitoring required

Fluvoxamine:
- Not proved effective by controlled study
- Open-label study indicates possible efficacy
- To minimize side effects, low-dose therapy is recommended
- Initiate dose at 25 mg at bedtime for three days
- Increase dose every three to four days until a maximum of 200 mg/day is achieved
- Give twice daily for daily doses of 75 mg or greater, with the larger dose given at bedtime
- Experimental
- Careful monitoring required

Table 5.8

Dosage and Administration of Fluoxetine, Sertraline, Paroxetine, and Fluvoxamine in OCD and Conditions with Obsessive-Compulsive Symptoms (i.e., Trichotillomania)

Fluoxetine:
- Effective treatment
- Combination therapy with clomipramine may enhance efficacy, decrease doses of both, and minimize side effect in treatment refractory OCD
- Monitor closely for possible increased risk of fluoxetine side effects (i.e., akathisia)

(Continued)

Table 5.8

(Continued)

- Start with fluoxetine 20 mg q.o.d. and clomipramine 25 mg
- If no response after 10–14 days, increase fluoxetine to 20 mg and clomipramine to 50 mg: may, after 10–14 days, increase fluoxetine to 20 mg b.i.d. if no response
- Carefully monitor clomipramine levels and signs of toxicity
- If clomipramine contraindicated, start with fluoxetine 20 mg q.o.d. and increase every 10–14 days to a maximum daily dose of 80 mg/day, i.e., 20 mg q.i.d.

Sertraline:

- Not known to be effective
- May be effective in adults
- Controlled study is necessary before this can be recommended for routine use

Paroxetine:

- Not known to be effective
- Not recommended for routine use

Fluvoxamine:

- Controlled study shows efficacy
- To minimize side effects, low-dose therapy is recommended
- Initiate dose at 25 mg at bedtime for three days
- Increase dose every three to four days until a maximum of 200 mg/day is achieved
- Give twice daily for daily doses of 75 mg or greater, with the larger dose given at bedtime
- Experimental
- Careful monitoring required

Trazodone

Trazodone is an atypical antidepressant that is chemically unrelated to the TCAs, and differs from TCAs in having almost no anticholinergic side effects. In adults, this agent has been used primarily to treat depression, although recent experience demonstrates its potential value in other areas (i.e., OCD) as well. Trazodone is best known for its sedative effect, and is often chosen when insomnia or other sleep disturbance is prominent.

Table 5.9

Dosage and Administration of Fluoxetine, Sertraline, Paroxetine, and Fluvoxamine in ADHD

Fluoxetine:
- No controlled studies documenting efficacy
- One open-label study suggests may be effective
- Only use after other standard medications fail
- Start with doses 20 mg q.o.d.
- If no improvement after 7 to 10 days, increase dose by 20 mg every 7 to 10 days until symptom relief or maximum dose of 80 mg/day (i.e., 20 mg q.i.d.)
- Careful monitoring required

Sertraline, Paroxetine, and Fluvoxamine:
- No controlled or open-label studies demonstrating efficacy
- Not recommended for use until further studied

Table 5.10

Dosage and Administration of Fluoxetine, Sertraline, Paroxetine, and Fluvoxamine in Self-Injurious Behavior

Fluoxetine:
- No controlled studies showing efficacy
- Anecdotal and open-label case studies indicate potential role
- Should only be used after nonchemical restraint found to be unsuccessful
- Need to start with very low doses and increase very gradually because of possible increased sensitivity of these patients to side effects
- Starting doses of 5 mg/day are suggested
- If no improvement, can increase dose by 5 mg every 10–14 days until symptom relief or toxicity
- Should not exceed 80 mg (i.e., 20 mg q.i.d.)
- Monitor closely for efficacy versus toxicity

Sertraline, Paroxetine, and Fluvoxamine:
- No controlled or open-label studies showing efficacy
- Not recommended for use until further studied

It is very effective in improving sleep quality, increasing total sleep time, and decreasing the number of nighttime awakenings.[27]

See Tables 5.11 and 5.12.

Priapism

Males taking trazodone must be told to report any prolonged erections immediately. The occurrence of priapism constitutes a medical emergency and the immediate discontinuation of trazodone is warranted.

Overdose/Toxicity

One advantage of trazodone is its relative lack of toxicity in overdose. There have been no reported lethal overdoses when trazodone was taken alone. However, fatalities have occurred when trazodone was taken with other drugs, and thus it is important to ask the patient and family what other drugs were ingested. Urine and serum drug screens are also necessary.

See Table 5.13.

Bupropion

Bupropion is an atypical antidepressant unrelated to the TCAs. In adults, it has been approved by FDA only for MDD, and it has not been approved for use in patients under 18 years of age. ADHD is the only disorder in this population where some evidence for bupropion's efficacy exists. It has few anticholinergic effects, and does not alter cardiac conduction or cause orthostasis.

Attention-Deficit/Hyperactivity Disorder

Bupropion was used to treat 30 prepubertal children with diagnoses of ADHD in a double-blind, placebo-controlled study, and was found to be safe and effective.[28] Several clinicians have found that children with prominent conduct disorder symptoms responded especially well to bupropion.[29] Optimal doses ranged from 3 to 7 mg/kg/day (100 to 250 mg/day).

Major Depressive Disorder

In adults, bupropion has been found to be as effective as standard antidepressant therapies in the treatment of MDD. There are no data on children and adolescents.

Table 5.11

Pharmacokinetics of Atypical Antidepressants

Generic Name (Brand Name)	Peak Plasma Concentrations (hours)	Plasma Half-Life (hours)	Metabolism and Excretion	Comments
Trazodone (Desyrel)	1–2	6–11	Liver—active metabolite *m*-chlorophenylpiperazine; excreted by kidneys	Inhibits serotonin reuptake; no anticholinergic effects
Bupropion (Wellbutrin)	2	8–24	Liver—metabolites hydroxybupropion and threohydrobupropion; excreted in urine	Hydroxybupropion concentrations > 1,250 ng/ml associated with lack of clinical response
Nefazodone (Serzone)	1	2–4	Liver—hydroxynefazodone, *m*-chlorophenylpiperazine, triazole-dione; excreted in urine	Serotonergic effects; sedative actions
Venlafaxine (Effexor)	2–3	3–4	Liver—o-desmethylvenlafaxine; excreted in urine	A mixed NE and 5-HT uptake inhibitor

Table 5.12

Side Effects of Trazodone

Common:
• Sedation
• Orthostasis (in adults, children?)
• Dizziness
• Headache
• Nausea/vomiting
Rare but Important:
• Priapism
No Cardiac, Anticholinergic Side Effects

Table 5.13

Trazodone Drug Interactions

Increases Serum Levels:
• Digoxin
• Phenytoin
• CNS depressants

See Table 5.14.

Contraindications

Bulimia /Anorexia Nervosa

A current or prior diagnosis of bulimia or anorexia nervosa contraindicates the use of bupropion. A higher incidence of seizures has been reported when bupropion was administered to these patients.

Patients on MAOIs

Bupropion should not be prescribed for patients on MAOIs. The patient should be off the MAOI for at least two weeks prior to the initiation of bupropion therapy.

Table 5.14

Contraindications to Bupropion Therapy for Children and Adolescents

Absolute:
- Known hypersensitivity
- Pregnancy
- On MAOI
- Past or current history of bulimia or anorexia nervosa
- Seizure disorder
- Organic brain disease
- History of head trauma
- CNS tumor
- EEG abnormalities
- Recent withdrawal from benzodiazepines or alcohol

Relative:
- Concomitant administration of psychotropics known to lower seizure threshold
- Hepatic disease
- Renal disease

Seizure Disorder
We recommend that bupropion be avoided for children and adolescents with seizure disorders until more is known about the medication.

Organic Brain Disease
Because of its significantly increased association with seizures, we do not recommend using bupropion for children and adolescents with a history of head trauma, CNS tumor, or other organic brain disease. Any EEG abnormalities probably contraindicate its use at this time, although consultation with a neurologist is advised.

We do not recommend bupropion for patients who have recently withdrawn from benzodiazepines or alcohol, because of its increased association with seizures.

Seizures
Seizures are the side effect of most concern with bupropion.

Table 5.15

Side Effects of Bupropion Therapy

• Seizures
• Agitation
• Weight loss
• Headache
• Nausea
• Upper respiratory complaints
Does Not:
• Impair cognition
• Cause daytime sleepiness
• Cause orthostasis
• Cause anticholinergic effect
• Cause weight gain
• Have cardiac effects

See Table 5.15.

Overdose

Bupropion is significantly safer than the TCAs when taken in overdose. Overdoses of bupropion when taken alone have not been fatal.

Abuse

There is no evidence that bupropion results in an increase in physical and psychological dependence.

Drug Interactions

Bupropion does cross the placenta, and so should not be prescribed during pregnancy. Thus, a pregnancy test and evaluation for adequate contraceptive use is essential for all females of child-bearing age.

See Table 5.16.

When children and adolescents are treated with bupropion, they should be monitored at each visit, by observation and history, for any involuntary movements/tics. Whenever the dose is increased, it is important to check blood pressure, pulse, height, and weight.

Table 5.16

Drug Interactions with Bupropion

Acute Toxicity may be Increased By:
• MAOIs
Increases Adverse Experiences When Administered Concurrently with:
• Levodopa
Use Caution When Administering with:
• Drug metabolized by liver
• Phenytoin
• Barbiturates
• Carbamazepine
• Cimetidine

See Table 5.17.

Nefazodone

Nefazodone is a synthetic phenylpiperazine compound that is similar to trazodone. It is a selective antagonist postsynaptically and inhibits the reuptake of serotonin at the central 5-HT$_2$ receptors. It has no significant affinity for the following receptors: alpha-2-adrenergic and beta-adrenergic, 5-HT$_{1A}$, cholinergic, dopaminergic, or benzodiazepine. There are three major metabolites: hydroxynefazodone, which possesses a pharmacologic profile similar to that of nefazodone; meta-chlorophenylpiperazine, which has some properties similar to those of the parent compound, but has agonistic activity at the serotonergic receptor; and triazole-dione, which has yet to be characterized.

Nefazodone is rapidly absorbed after oral administration and produces peak blood concentrations in one hour postingestion. It has a half-life of two to four hours, while hydroxynefazodone and meta-chlorophenylpiperazine have half-lives of one and a half to four hours and four to eight hours respectively.

The drug is extensively metabolized by the liver, has 20% absolute bioavailability, and with less than 1% excreted

Table 5.17

Dosage and Administration of Bupropion for Children and Adolescents

---

ADHD:
- Some open-label and controlled studies show possible efficacy
- Start with test dose 100 mg/day
- If this is tolerated well, increase dose to 100 mg b.i.d.
- Do not administer individual doses >150 mg
- Increase doses by 100 mg every 7 to 10 days to a maximum of 450 mg/day
- Doses of 150 mg should be given at least six hours apart

MDD:
- No studies demonstrating efficacy
- Adult studies show effectiveness
- Use adult guidelines
- Only use if standard agents fail (i.e., TCAs, fluoxetine)
- Start with dose 100 mg/day
- If tolerated, increase dose to 100 mg b.i.d.
- Increase dose by 100 mg every 7 to 10 days until symptoms relieved, toxicity, or maximum dose of 450 mg/day
- Do not administer individual dose of more than 150 mg
- Give doses of 150 mg at least six hours apart

---

unchanged in the urine. After oral administration of radiolabeled nefazodone, approximately 55% of the administered radioactivity was detected in urine and 20 to 30% in feces. Nefazodone is extensively bound to human plasma proteins (>99%) at concentrations of 25 to 2,500 ng/ml.

The average effective dose range in adults is 300 to 600 mg/day in two divided doses. The initial dose is 200 mg/day, with increases in increments of 100 to 200 mg/day every seven days. All dosages should be decreased by 50% in elderly patients.

Venlafaxine

Venlafaxine is a phenylethylamine derivative. It inhibits the reuptake of three neurotransmitters, norepinephrine, serotonin, and dopamine. The major metabolite is *o*-desmethylvenlafaxine, which is as potent as the parent drug in blocking reuptake and receptor binding, and is usually present in concentrations that exceed those of the parent compound.

Venlafaxine is rapidly absorbed after oral administration and produces peak blood concentrations in two to three hours. It has a half-life of three to four hours and its major metabolite has a half-life of about 10 hours.

The drug is extensively metabolized by the liver and approximately 85% of a single dose is excreted in the urine within 72 hours. Unlike the SSRIs that are highly protein bound, venlafaxine is only weakly bound, 25 to 30%.

The dosage for adults is 75 to 350 mg/day by mouth.

References

1. Bardeleben, U.V., Steiger, A., Gerken, A., et al. (1989). Effects of fluoxetine upon pharmacoendocrine and sleep-EEG parameters in normal controls. *Int Clin Psychopharmacol, 4*, 1–5.
2. Emslie, G.J., Rush, A.J., Weinberg, W.A. A double-blind, randomized placebo-controlled trial of fluoxoetine in depressed children and adolescents. *Arch Gen Psychiatry*, in press.
3. Berman, I., Sapers, B.L., Saltzman, C. (1992). Sertraline: A new sertonergic antidepressant. *Hosp Community Psychiatry, 43*, 671–672.
4. Cohn, C.K., Shrivastava, R., Mendels, J., et al. (1990). Double-blind, multicenter comparison of sertraline and amitriptyline in elderly depressed patients. *J Clin Psychiatry, 51* (suppl. B), 28–33.
5. Doogan, D.P., Calliard, V. (1988). Sertraline: A new antidepressant. *J Clin Psychiatry, 49* (suppl.), 46–51.
6. Reimherr, F.W., Chouinard, G., Cohn, C.K., et al. (1990). Antidepressant efficacy of sertraline: A double-blind, placebo- and amitriptyline-controlled, multicenter comparison study in outpatients with major depression. *J Clin Psychiatry, 51* (suppl. B), 18–27.
7. Benfield, P., Heel, R.C., Lewis, S.P. (1986). Fluoxetine: A review of its pharmacodynamic and pharmacokinetic properties, and therapeutic efficacy in depressive illness. *Drugs, 32*, 481–508.
8. Emslie, G., Rush, A., Weonberg, W., et al. (1995). Efficacy of fluoxetine in depressed children and adolescents. Presented at the 42nd Annual Meeting of the American Academy of Child and Adolescent Psychiatry, New Orleans, LA.
9. Fava, M., Rosenbaum, J.F. (1991). Suicidality and fluoxetine: Is there a relationship? *J Clin Psychiatry, 52*, 108–111.

10. Simeon, J.G., Thatte, S., Wiggins, D. (1990). Treatment of adolescent obsessive-compulsive disorder with a clomipramine–fluoxetine combination, *Psychopharmacol Bull, 26,* 285–290.

11. Chouinard, G., Goodman, W., Greist, J., et al. (1990). Results of a double-blind placebo-controlled trial of a new serotonin uptake inhibitor, sertraline, in the treatment of obsessive compulsive disorder. *Psychopharmacol Bull, 26,* 279–284.

12. McDougle, C.J., Price, L.H., Volkmar, F.R., et al. (1992). Clomipramine in autism: Preliminary evidence of efficacy. *J Am Acad Child Adolesc Psychiatry, 31,* 746–750.

13. Kennedy, S.H., Piran, N., Garfinkel, P.E. (1985). Monoamine oxidase inhibitor therapy for anorexia nervosa and bulimia: A preliminary trial of isocarboxazid. *J Clin Psychopharmacol, 5,* 279–285.

14. Pope, H.G., Hudson, J.I., Jonas, J.M., et al. (1983). Bulimia treatment with imipramine: A double-blind placebo-controlled study. *Am J Psychiatry, 14,* 554–558.

15. Mitchell, J.E., Groat, R. (1984). A placebo-controlled double-blind trial of amitriptyline in bulimia. *J Clin Psychopharmacol, 4,* 186–193.

16. Hughes, P.L., Wall, L.A., Cunningham, C.J., et al. (1986). Treating bulimia with desipramine. *Arch Gen Psychiatry, 43,* 182–186.

17. Walsh, B.T., Stewart, J.M., Roose, S.P., et al. (1984). Treatment of bulimia with phenelzine. *Arch Gen Psychiatry, 41,* 1105–1109.

18. Arana, G.W., Hyman, S.E. (Eds.) (1991). *Handbook of Psychiatric Drug Therapy* (2nd ed.) (pp. 38–78). Boston: Little Brown.

19. Riddle, M.A., King, R.A., Hardin, M.T., et al. (1990). Behavioral side effects of fluoxetine in children and adolescents. *J Child Adolesc Psychopharmacol, 1,* 193–198.

20. Cole, J.O., Bodkin, J.A. (1990). Antidepressant drug side effects. *J Clin Psychiatry, 51* (suppl. 1), 21–26.

21. Herman, J.B., Brotman, A.W., Pollack, M.H., et al. (1990). Fluoxetine-induced sexual dysfunction. *J Clin Psychiatry, 51,* 25.

22. Kaplan, H.I., Sadock, B.J. (1991). Biological therapies. In H.I. Kaplan, B.J. Sadock (Eds.), *Synopsis of Psychiatry* (6th ed.) (p. 650). Baltimore: Williams & Wilkins.

23. Settle, E.C., Jr., Settle, G.P. (1984). A case of mania associated with fluoxetine. *Am J Psychiatry, 141,* 280–281.

24. Turner, S.M., Jacob, R.G., Beidel, D., et al. (1985). A second case of mania associated with fluoxetine (letter). *Am J Psychiatry, 142,* 274–275.

25. Hon, D., Preskorn, S.H. (1989). Mania during fluoxetine treatment for recurrent depression (letter). *Am J Psychiatry, 146,* 1638–1639.

26. *Physicians' Desk Reference* (50th ed.) (1996). Oradell, NJ: Medical Economics.

27. Mouret, J., Cemoine, P., Minuit, M.P., et al. (1988). Effects of trazodone on the sleep of depressed subjects: A polysomnographic study. *Psychopharmacology*, *95*, 537.

28. Clay, T.H., Gaultieri, C.T., Evans, R.W., et al. (1988). Clinical and neuropsychological effects of the novel antidepressant bupropion. *Psychopharmacol Bull*, *24*, 143–148.

29. Simeon, J.G., Ferguson, H.B., Fleet, J.W. (1986). Bupropion effects in attention deficit and conduct disorders. *Can J Psychiatry*, *31*, 581–585.

C h a p t e r   6

Monoamine Oxidase Inhibitors (MAOIs)

A tremendous amount of research has demonstrated the effectiveness of monoamine oxidase inhibitors (MAOIs) for a variety of psychiatric disorders. However, in practice these agents are difficult and risky to administer. With the widening selection of antidepressants now available, MAOIs are used infrequently in adults, and quite rarely in children.

All drugs in this class inhibit, either reversibly or irreversibly, the enzyme monoamine oxidase (MAO). In addition to its central role in the metabolism of neurotransmitters, MAO also metabolizes dietary tyramine, the interruption of which can lead to a dangerous hypertensive crisis. Therefore, use of an MAOI requires strict adherence to a low-tyramine diet. This liability alone is sufficient to recommend against the use of MAOIs for children and adolescents, where strict dietary control is usually impossible. The synthesis of several new MAOIs that are less sensitive to tyramine has prompted renewed academic interest and requires that clinicians remain familiar with these agents, but does not change the fact that they currently have little application in child and adolescent psychiatric disorders.

Two main MAOI compounds are marketed in the United States for psychiatric indications: phenelzine (Nardil) and tranylcypromine (Parnate). Several others, however, are in use internationally or under investigation (Table 6.1). The most important chemical property of these agents is whether they are nonreversible (require dietary restrictions) or reversible (involve

Table 6.1

Current MAOIs

Nonselective	
Iproniazid (Marsalid)	Irreversible
Isocarboxazid (Marplan)	Irreversible
Phenelzine (Nardil)	Irreversible
Tranylcypromine (Parnate)	Irreversible*
Selective MAO-A	
Clorgyline	Irreversible†
Moclobemide	Reversible
Selective MAO-B	
Selegiline (Eldepryl)	Irreversible†
Pargyline (Eutonyl)	Irreversible†
*Partially reversible in vitro. †Nonselective at higher doses.	

no dietary restrictions). Both currently available drugs are nonreversible MAOIs.

Indications

General Issues Regarding Children and Adolescents

Guidelines for the use of MAOIs exist only for adults, for whom they have been effective in the treatment of depression, anxiety, and other disorders. Although the same clinical indications characterize children, there have been very few controlled studies of the use of MAOIs in this population. However, since selective, reversible agents, such as moclobemide, may become available in the United States, the risk factors that traditionally limited the prescription of MAOIs for children may become less relevant.

See Table 6.2.

Major Depression
MAOIs appear to be as effective as the heterocyclic compounds for classic major depression.[1] There have been no systematic comparisons of MAOIs with the newer antidepressants (SSRIs, buproprion, etc.).[2]

Table 6.2

Psychiatric Indications (in Adults) for MOAIs

Established	Major and "atypical" depression Depressive disorders refractory to TCAs and SSRIs Panic disorder with or without agoraphobia Social phobia/agoraphobia without panic
Experimental	ADHD Childhood depression (<16 years) Anorexia and bulimia Separation anxiety/school phobia

Atypical Depression

In the broadest sense, "atypical" refers to any depressive disorder that does not exhibit the classic signs of endogenous or melancholic depression. The most common manifestation of atypical depression is a subtype of major depression with "reversed" neurovegetative signs: weight gain rather than loss, hypersomnia rather than insomnia, mood reactivity, and mood worsening in the evening rather than the morning. This subtype of depression has been thought to respond preferentially to MAOI therapy and is more common in adolescents.[1]

Child and Adolescent Depression

Very little has been written about the use of MAOIs for childhood and adolescent depression, owing to the high associated risks. Nevertheless, the two extant studies of MAOIs in child and adolescent depression are favorable.[3,4]

Panic Disorder

Reports of the successful treatment of panic attacks with MAOIs date back to the late 1950s, with more recent studies reporting positive results.[5] Agoraphobia and related phobic states likewise respond well to MAOIs—in some studies, better than to benzodiazepines.[6]

Attention-Deficit/Hyperactivity Disorder

Zametkin and associates[7] have compared psychostimulants to several medications that alter catecholamine metabolism as treatments for ADHD. In a double-blind crossover study of MAOIs in 14 boys with ADHD, both clorgyline (irreversible MAO-A inhibitor) and tranylcypromine "so closely paralleled dextroamphetamine that the treating physician could not distinguish between them."[7] Although MAOIs certainly cannot be recommended for the routine outpatient management of ADHD, these data do raise hopes that reversible MAOIs may offer an alternative to psychostimulants. Moclobemide has, in fact, been used successfully in an open trial of 11 ADHD patients who had failed or were intolerant of stimulant treatment.

Contraindications

MAOI treatment is contraindicated in a variety of circumstances, most of which relate to concurrent medical illness or pharmacologic treatment. It is advisable to test the ability to comply with dietary restrictions by reviewing a detailed log of food and beverage for two weeks prior to instituting therapy (see Clinical Practice). Additional contraindications are given in Table 6.3.

If the patient has been treated with any serotonergic agent (including paroxetine, sertraline, buspirone, trazodone, doxepin,

Table 6.3

Contraindications to Treatment with MAOIs

- Inability to maintain dietary restrictions
- Concurrent use of any sympathomimetic agents known to react with MAOIs
- Concurrent use with other drugs with MAOI activity
- Concurrent use of SSRIs
- Pheochromocytoma
- Preexisting liver disease
- Preexisting cerebrovascular disease or untreated hypertension
- Impending surgery requiring general or local anesthesia
- Asthma when sympathomimetic bronchodilators are unavoidable

and tricyclic antidepressants), a 7- to 14-day "washout" period is required before starting an MAOI (see Drug Interactions below). A 14-day washout is similarly necessary when changing from one MAOI to another. Fluoxetine (Prozac) has an extended elimination half-life requiring at least a five-week washout period.

Concurrent use of sympathomimetics, either prescribed, in over-the-counter preparations, or through excessive caffeine intake, are contraindicated (Table 6.4).

Table 6.4

Medications That are Contraindicated with MAOI Therapy

Degree of Caution	Medication	Comments and Examples
Common Agents That are Absolutely Contraindicated	Sympathomimetic amines	Prescription (Rx)— Amphetamine and epinephrine analogs; Non-Rx— ephedrine, pseudoephedrine, phenylephrine, and phenylethylamine
	Dextromethorphan	OTC—present in Dristan, Comtrex, and many others; acts via serotonin reuptake blockade
	SSRIs	Rx—fluoxetine, sertraline, paroxetine, etc. May produce serotonin syndrome (see text)
	Hypoglycemic agents	Rx—potentiates hypoglycemia
	L-Dopa, methyldopa	Rx—enhances pressor effect. Dopamine present in some food
	Reserpine	Rx—similar to serotonin syndrome
	Tryptophan	Rx—serotonin precursor

(Continued)

Table 6.4

(Continued)

Anesthetic Agents to be Avoided	Narcotic analgesics	Primarily meperidine and other 5-HT blockers, but may also prolong action of morphine and barbiturates
	Ketamine	Theoretical risk of cardiovascular toxicity
	Suxamethonium	May prolong or increase neuromuscular blockade
	Local anesthetics	Avoid epinephrine, norepinephrine, cocaine, and analogs
Agents Causing Adverse Reactions in Rare Cases	Amantadine	Acts as a dopamine agonist; may produce hypertension
	Chloral hydrate	Hypertension reported, mechanism unknown
	Droperidol	Hypotension reported
	Fenfluramine	Delirium reported, mechanism unknown
	Guanethidine	May produce hypertension
Agents to be Used with Caution	TCAs Anticholinergics	See guidelines in textbook Potentiation reported in humans, hyperthermia in animals
	Benzodiazepines	Reports of edema; probably safe
	Caffeine	Hypertension and agitation with excessive intake

Side Effects

Hypertensive Crisis

A discussion of the side effects of MAOIs inevitably focuses on the so-called "cheese effect", or the hypertensive reaction produced by dietary tyramine in patients treated with irreversible MAOIs. Even when patients adhere to dietary restrictions, the incidence of hypertensive crisis is around 3.3%. Typically, a hypertensive crisis presents with severe occipital headache, palpitations, neck stiffness, nausea, vomiting, diaphoresis, pupillary dilation, photophobia, and chest pain. Hypertension has, in rare cases, been severe enough to cause intracranial bleeding and death.

The Serotonin Syndrome

A well-established interaction has been described between serotonin reuptake inhibitors and MAOIs, referred to as the serotonergic syndrome or central excitatory syndrome. The clinical features include mental status changes (confusion, agitation, hypomania), myoclonus, hyperreflexia, tremor, ataxia, diaphoresis, fever, and autonomic dysregulation.[8]

Cardiovascular Effects

MAOI therapy is associated with both decreased and increased resting blood pressure (RBP). The decrease in RBP is most notable in subjects who were hypertensive at baseline. Orthostatic hypotension is reportedly common.

Manic Symptoms

Although a well-known reaction to heterocyclic antidepressants, mania caused by MAOIs was recognized rather late. Cases have also been reported of mania induced by combining MAOIs and TCAs in depressed bipolar patients.

General Effects

Less common adverse effects include insomnia, impotence, edema, weight gain, elevated hepatic enzymes, and overstimulation (jitteriness, tremors, twitching). Psychotic symptoms may emerge or be exacerbated in rare cases.

Overdose

Much of the information on MAOI overdose comes not from the psychiatric literature, but from oncology reports, where MAOI agents are used in antineoplastic regimens. If the patient has also ingested a source of tyramine or sympathomimetics, an overdosage is treated much like a hypertensive crisis (see below). However, death has been reported from MAOI overdose alone. Periods of deep sedation may alternate with unrestrainable agitation and autonomic dysregulation. Specific symptoms may include drowsiness, dizziness, mental status changes (agitation, hyperactivity, confusion, or psychosis), headache, seizures, and coma.

Drug Interactions

The list of medications that are incompatible with MAOIs is extensive and includes many agents available as over-the-counter products. These are detailed in Table 6.4.

Clinical Practice

The authors do not recommend the use of MAOIs in a typical outpatient pediatric practice, and guidelines for children and adolescents are virtually nonexistent. However, in the event that a child must be placed on an irreversible MAOI, or has been prescribed an MAOI by another clinician, we suggest the following methods.

Education about and adherence to dietary and medication restrictions are necessary before starting MAOI therapy. A verbal discussion of restrictions is not sufficient. It is advisable to provide well-organized and simply written handouts, which may be posted at home and referred to frequently. Since a washout period of 7–14 days (more for fluoxetine) is required when changing from another antidepressant to an MAOI (see discussion above), this is the best time to test the patient's ability to comply with dietary restrictions. If the patient and family are unable to keep an accurate and compliant dietary log for the two weeks prior to therapy, then MAOI therapy is probably not possible. (See Table 6.5).

Dosing is conservative, even for older children, starting with one tablet of phenelzine (15 mg) or tranylcypromine (10 mg) daily, rather than the three recommended for adults. Dose increases should not be more frequent than every 14 days, since maximal MAO inhibition is achieved in 7–14 days. In one trial, an average phenelzine dose of 15 mg twice daily was well tolerated by children ages 9 to 15 years.[3]

Management of Specific Side Effects

Hypertensive Crisis

Even with good compliance, patients may forget about certain forbidden foods or inadvertently ingest foods that they did not realize were rich in tyramine. Extensive premedication counseling is necessary so that the symptoms of a pressor

Table 6.5

Dietary Restrictions with MAOI Therapy

Dietary Guidelines	Tyramine* (mg/30 g)	Comments and Examples
Not Permitted		
Cheese, aged, overripe, or spoiled	1.0–65.0	Blue, cheddar, Gruyere
Smoked, pickled, or unfresh fish	0–99.0	Caviar, anchovies, herring
Fermented dry sausage	3.0–45	Pepperoni, salami, summer sausage
semidry sausage	~2.6	Bologna
Beer imported or import-style ale	0.05–0.4	Twelve ounces of American-style beer contain about 1 mg
American style beer	0.05–0.1	tyramine
Red wine, sherry, liqueurs	0.05–0.4	Especially Chianti (0.76 mg/30 ml)
Beef or chicken liver	0–0.3	May be acceptable if very fresh
Meat extracts	2.9–9.1	Bovril, Marmite, some dry soup bases
Yeast extracts and supplements	2.0–68.0	Regular bakery products are permitted
Sauerkraut	0.6–2.9	Testing done on German products
Unfresh or overripe protein-rich foods	Varies	Leftover meats and expired dairy products
Broad beans (e.g., fava beans)	NA	Contains dopamine rather than tyramine
Green banana or banana peel	0.2–2.0	Peel also contains dopamine
Permitted in Limited Amounts		
Processed American cheeses	0–1.5	Up to 1.5 mg of tyramine in a single slice (1 ounce) of American cheese

(Continued)

Table 6.5

(Continued)

Avocado	0–0.7	Higher levels in overripe fruit and guacamole
Bananas, fresh	0–0.2	Avoid overripe fruit and peel
Soy sauce and variants	~0.05	Safe unless used in very large amounts
Peanuts and other nuts	?	No documentation of tyramine content
Raspberries, fresh or in jams	~0.3–2.9	Safe in very small servings
White wine and distilled spirits	?	No documentation of tyramine content
Chocolate	NA	Contains phenylethylamine
Need not be Restricted		
Yogurt, sour cream, cream cheese, cottage cheese	0–0.3	Avoid homemade or homemade styles and consume very fresh products
Fresh fish and meats	ND	Do not allow spoilage
Fresh fruits (except raspberries)	ND	
Figs and raisins	ND	Canned figs may contain tyramine
Most dried soups and bouillon	ND	

*Figures based on 1-ounce (30 g or 30 ml) portions. Up to 6 mg of tyramine may be ingested safely while taking therapeutic doses of MAOIs.
Abbreviations: ND—no detectable amount of tyramine; NA—not applicable, contains other pressor agents.

response (headache, diaphoresis, stiff neck, nausea, and vomiting) will be promptly recognized and immediate medical attention will be available. Patients in remote locations or without access to emergency medical services should probably not receive MAOIs, since hospitalization may be required. Chlorpromazine has been used as a short-term treatment measure, leading to the recommendation that several 50-mg tablets (25 mg for children) be provided for patients to take if symptoms appear, especially if they will be temporarily away from medical care.[9] *Dietary and medication restrictions must be maintained for two weeks after discontinuation of an MAOI* and during the treatment of a hypertensive reaction.

Serotonin Syndrome

If a serotonin syndrome is suspected, any possible offending medications must be discontinued promptly. Frequently, hospitalization and supportive treatment are needed. Myoclonus, seizures, and agitation have been reported and may require pharmacologic treatment.

Cardiovascular Effects

Hypotension is often tolerable or may be managed with the use of increased fluids and salts. Yet, a number of patients will be unable to continue MAOI therapy owing to symptomatic hypotension. Of course, pressor agents are to be completely avoided.

How to Withdraw Medication

Withdrawal symptoms have ranged from anxiety and agitation to frank psychosis. Gradual discontinuation of the medication is recommended. Regardless of how the medication is discontinued, MOA activity is suppressed for up to two weeks after the last dose, necessitating full compliance with dietary and medication restrictions during that period.

References

1. Ravaris, C.L., Robinson, D.S., Ives, J.O., et al. (1980). Phenelzine and amitriptyline in the treatment of depression. A comparison of present and past studies. *Arch Gen Psychiatry, 37*, 1075–1080.
2. Gabelic, I., Moll, E. (1990). Moclobemide (Ro 11-1163) versus desipramine in the treatment of endogenous depression. *Acta Psychiatr Scand, 360 (suppl.)*, 44–45.
3. Frommer, E.A. (1967). Treatment of childhood depression with antidepressant drugs. *BMJ, 1*, 729–732.
4. Ryan, N.D., Puig-Antich, J., Rabinovich, H., et al. (1988). MAOIs in adolescent major depression unresponsive to tricyclic antidepressants. *J Am Acad Child Adolesc Psychiatry, 27*, 755–758.
5. Buigues, J., Vallejo, J. (1987). Therapeutic response to phenelzine in patients with panic disorder and agoraphobia with panic attacks. *J Clin Psychiatry, 48*, 55–59.

6. Gelernter, C.S., Uhde, T.W., Cimbolic, P., et al. (1991). Cognitive-behavioral and pharmacological treatments of social phobia. A controlled study. *Arch Gen Psychiatry*, *48*, 938–945.
7. Zametkin, A., Rapoport, J.L., Murphy, D.L., et al. (1985). Treatment of hyperactive children with monoamine oxidase inhibitors. I. Clinical efficacy. *Arch Gen Psychiatry*, *42*, 962–966.
8. Sternbach, H. (1991). The serotonin syndrome. *Am J Psychiatry*, *148*, 705–713.
9. Kaplan, H.I., Sadock, B.J. (1991). *Synopsis of Psychiatry* (pp. 382, 656–667). Baltimore: Williams & Wilkins.

Antipsychotic Agents

Of all the medicines used for psychiatric illness, antipsychotics are the most important historically. These agents (also called neuroleptics or major tranquilizers) virtually emptied the custodial institutions which were infamous as providers of mental health care prior to 1950. The use of antipsychotics in children has been well studied, despite the fact that these agents bear considerable risks.

Seven agents have FDA approval for psychiatric indications in children younger than 12 years. Although they can be quite effective, antipsychotics should not be considered for children and adolescents unless serious psychopathology is present and is greatly impairing normal function. This caution is based on the potentially serious neurologic and developmental effects of antipsychotics, which are discussed in this chapter.

Antipsychotic agents are chemically diverse and block a number of neuroreceptor sites, including dopamine, acetylcholine, serotonin, catecholamines, and histamine. Although their clinical potency correlates best with antidopamine properties, effects at other receptor sites are becoming increasingly important. For example, clozapine has emerged as one of the more effective antipsychotics for schizophrenia, and yet possesses relatively low antidopamine potency as compared with older agents.

Indications

Antipsychotics are indicated primarily for the treatment of psychosis, and their use for childhood psychosis parallels that

Table 7.1

Indications for Antipsychotic Therapy in Children and Adolescents

Recommended Uses:
• Schizophrenia and other psychoses
• Tourette's syndrome (when functional impairment is severe)
• Some acute drug intoxications
• Delirium
• Self-injurious behavior (when behavioral management has failed)
• Uncontrollable aggression
Not Recommended, but Sometimes Used for:
• Tourette's syndrome (when tics are intolerable)
• Nonpsychotic anxiety
• Severe behavioral disruption, or agitation, without aggression
• Autism, without a specific indication

for adults. Other indications are listed in Table 7.1. Yet it must be emphasized that even when those indications are clearly present, the decision to use antipsychotics in a particular child or adolescent must involve carefully weighing the risks of these medications against that individual's functional impairment and potential benefit.

Schizophrenia

After decades of diagnostic confusion, the term "childhood schizophrenia" is now reserved for cases in which adult symptom criteria are met, adjusting only for the developmental context of the child's symptoms.[1] Using this modern definition, the prevalence of schizophrenia in children under 13 years of age may be as low as 1.9 per 100,000.[2] In fact, most prepubescent children who present with the complaint of hallucinations are not schizophrenic and require no pharmacologic treatment.[3] The age of onset for schizophrenia is commonly late adolescence through young adulthood.

Once the diagnosis of schizophrenia has been established in a child or adolescent, the treatment guidelines parallel those established for adult schizophrenia. All commonly prescribed antipsychotics have been found superior to placebo in treating the positive symptoms of schizophrenia.[4] Maintenance treatment with neuroleptics is likewise superior to placebo in the prevention of relapse. Therefore, the main tasks facing the clinician are choosing the most appropriate agent, managing common side effects, and monitoring for serious adverse reactions, each of which is described below.

Positive and Negative Symptoms
The manifestations of schizophrenia classically have been divided into positive symptoms (hallucinations, delusions, ideas of reference, and formal thought disorder) and negative symptoms (withdrawal, flattening of affect, amotivation, and apathy). While antipsychotic agents are unequivocally effective against the former, the question of whether classic agents treat, aggravate, or have any effect on negative symptoms remains undecided. Modern agents, such as clozapine and risperidone, are felt to be more effective for negative symptoms, possibly due to their enhanced serotonergic activity.

Transient Psychoses
Transient psychotic symptoms can be seen in several clinical conditions: affective disorders (major depression and bipolar disorder), drug abuse or overdose, nonschizophrenic paranoid disorders, and organic mental disorders. Paranoid disorders are rarely diagnosed in children, but drug abuse, affective disorders, and organic mental disorders are encountered. Although the use of neuroleptics in such cases has not been systematically studied, case studies and clinical practice have demonstrated their effectiveness under certain conditions.

Drug Abuse or Overdose
Neuroleptics are useful for treating acute intoxication with certain psychoactive drugs, especially hallucinogens and phencyclidine (PCP). High-potency agents (e.g., haloperidol) in low doses are preferable in these cases to avoid anticholinergic effects. Low-potency agents should be used with caution because of their anticholinergic properties. However, neuroleptics are contraindicated for sedative overdose and during withdrawal states, as they may further depress consciousness or mask life-threatening withdrawal symptoms. See Chapter 14 for further discussion of substance abuse treatment.

Delirium

Delirium is distinguished from other cognitive disturbances by its relatively rapid onset, the presence of a fluctuating level of consciousness, and a suspected medical or neurologic cause. Diffuse background slowing on an EEG may help distinguish delirium from other mental syndromes, especially if a previous EEG is available for comparison. Pediatric causes include direct brain injury, CNS neoplasms, Addison's disease, Wilson's disease, hyper- or hypothyroidism, and other metabolic disorders. There have been no controlled studies of neuroleptics for delirium in children, but their use in adults is well documented. Low-dose haloperidol is favored because of its minimal anticholinergic activity.

Tourette's Syndrome

Of the several recognized tic disorders, only Tourette's syndrome is an approved indication for treatment with neuroleptic agents. Other disorders may mimic Tourette's, so care must be taken to diagnose the syndrome accurately. In addition, any psychostimulants must be discontinued, as they can greatly exacerbate tics.

Two antipsychotic agents are approved for use in Tourette's syndrome: haloperidol (Haldol) and pimozide (Orap). The effectiveness of each has been well demonstrated in placebo-controlled studies,[5] although pimozide may be better tolerated. Clonidine should be considered as a possible alternative to pimozide or haloperidol (see Chapter 11). Although less effective at controlling tics, it has fewer severe risks and may help comorbid behavioral problems.

Since these agents are unquestionably effective in reducing tics, the most important clinical question is whether reducing tics is necessary. Erenberg[6] estimates that with appropriate support and education, as many as 50% of Tourette's patients can tolerate tics, without significant functional compromise and without incurring the risks associated with neuroleptic therapy.

Pervasive Developmental Disorder

Autism and other pervasive developmental disorders are quite difficult to diagnose and treat effectively. Although antipsychotics are often used, the diagnosis of autism alone should not be considered an indication for antipsychotic therapy. No study has shown neuroleptics to be an effective treatment for the core symptoms of autism, although children with autism can and do display many of the other symptomatic indications for neuroleptic therapy. They may, for example, be more likely to display aggression and self-abuse than the normal population. Neuroleptics have been shown to reduce stereotypies (repetitive, self-stimulatory behaviors), aggression, and agitation in both autistic and nonautistic children. Therefore, the decision as to whether a neuroleptic is indicated and whether the risk of treatment is warranted should be made independently of the diagnosis of autism.

Attention-Deficit/Hyperactivity Disorder

This disorder is commonly managed with behavioral therapy and, if necessary, psychostimulants (Chapter 3). Refractory or atypical cases may be treated with heterocyclic antidepressants (Chapter 4), clonidine (Chapter 11), or other agents. Although neuroleptics generally are not considered for ADHD at all, they are nevertheless mentioned in most reviews of child psychopharmacology.

As with autistic disorder, neuroleptics are not indicated for ADHD alone, nor for its core symptoms. However, children with ADHD may occasionally display other symptomatic indications, such as severe aggression. Several placebo-controlled studies have reported improvement when neuroleptics were used alone or in combination with stimulants.[7,8] The use of antipsychotics in such cases is only justified when all other pharmacologic and behavioral measures have been exhausted and the clinician has evidence that the risks from the target behavior exceed the risks of neuroleptic therapy. Neuroleptics have been shown to hamper cognitive performance in hyperactive children and are, therefore, usually counterproductive to the goals of ADHD therapy.[9]

Nonspecific Behavioral Problems

Behavioral problems make up the bulk of child psychiatric referrals. Neuroleptics have been used in the treatment of behaviors that are dangerous, are severely disruptive to the child's development, and have failed to respond to behavioral or alternative pharmacologic measures.

Self-Injurious Behavior

Self-injurious behavior (SIB) is associated with a variety of developmental disorders. Pharmacologic intervention should be considered when the behavior is chronic, is severe enough to produce injury, and has failed behavioral treatment and other pharmacologic trials (e.g., stimulants, antidepressants, and anticonvulsants). Low-potency, sedating neuroleptics are typically used, although virtually every neuroleptic tested has shown some benefit.[10]

Aggression

Severe aggression that appears to be uncontrollable by the child is associated with many child psychiatric diagnoses, particularly developmental disorders. Pharmacologic treatment alone usually is not sufficient, but is often a valuable part of the broader treatment plan.[11] Short courses of neuroleptics are effective in reducing aggression across several diagnostic categories.[12] For the purposes of this discussion, the term "aggression" refers only to uncontrollable violent outbursts. Neuroleptics are not recommended for premeditated aggression associated with conduct disorder, gang-related behavior, and criminal activity.

For acute agitated aggression in the inpatient setting, the authors favor trying an intramuscular (IM) benzodiazepine (e.g., lorazepam 1 mg) or antihistamine (e.g., diphenhydramine 25–50 mg) before resorting to antipsychotics, especially for the first episode. These agents are discussed in Chapter 10. If the child fails to respond or becomes disinhibited with these agents, a sedating neuroleptic may be effective.

For chronic aggression in the outpatient setting, several medications should be tried before antipsychotics are prescribed. These include lithium, clonidine, beta-adrenergic blocking agents, buspirone, and anticonvulsants. Each of these is discussed elsewhere in this handbook. If neuroleptics must be used, we recommend starting with low doses of high-potency agents to minimize cognitive effects.

Nonaggressive agitation, such as encountered in developmental disorders, anxiety disorders, and situational reactions, has resulted in the use of sedating neuroleptics on a short-term basis. Specific behaviors may include restlessness, pacing, verbal disruption, or property destruction. Several antipsychotic agents are approved for such episodes of severe agitation, subsumed under the terms "severe behavioral disruption" and "nonpsychotic anxiety" (Table 7.1). Despite FDA approval of neuroleptics, the authors consider them to be a poor therapeutic choice unless the agitation is felt to be a manifestation of psychosis. In fact, such side effects as akathisia may exacerbate the condition.

Contraindications

The only absolute contraindications to the use of neuroleptics are type IV hypersensitivity, acute agranulocytosis, and current episodes of neuroleptic malignant syndrome (NMS). However, these agents should also be avoided in comatose or obtunded patients, patients who have received high doses of CNS depressants (such as narcotics or barbiturates), patients with a history of blood dyscrasias or bone marrow suppression (especially if related to neuroleptic use), and those with a subcortical brain injury with temperature dysregulation.

See Table 7.2.

Table 7.2

Contraindications to Antipsychotic Therapy

Definite
- Hypersensitivity to neuroleptics
- Agranulocytosis associated with neuroleptics
- NMS (acute)

Probable
- Comatose or obtunded patients
- Patients receiving high-dose CNS depressants
- Preexisting bone marrow suppression
- Subcortical temperature dysregulation

Relative
- History of NMS
- Pregnancy

Relative contraindications include pregnancy and previous NMS. While there is no proven risk to a fetus, animal studies suggest that these agents should be avoided in pregnancy when possible. How and when to restart an antipsychotic in a patient who has had a past episode of NMS is discussed below (see Adverse Reactions).

Side Effects and Adverse Reactions

Most antipsychotic side effects are related to specific neuroreceptors. Therefore, it may also be helpful to refer to Tables 7.3, 7.4, and 7.5 when reviewing side effects and when choosing a specific agent.

Extrapyramidal symptoms (EPS) are directly related to dopaminergic potency. The usual presentation is a parkinsonian syndrome of muscular rigidity (with or without cogwheeling), tremor, bradykinesia, masked facies, shuffling (festinating) gate, and drooling. Since these symptoms are relieved by anticholinergic agents, they are less common with neuroleptics that have anticholinergic properties.

Anticholinergic drugs used to treat EPS include both specific and nonspecific agents, many with significant antihistaminic activity as well. Among these are benztropine (Cogentin), biperiden (Akineton), and trihexyphenidyl (Artane).

Table 7.3

Side Effects of and Adverse Reactions to Antipsychotic Drugs

Short-term	Long-term	Idiosyncratic
• EPS	• Tardive dyskinesia	• NMS
• Acute dystonia	• Hyperprolactinemia	• Agranulocytosis
• Cardiac arrhythmias	• Hepatic toxicity	• Sudden death
• Anticholinergic symptoms	• Ocular pigmentation	
• Akathisia	• Photosensitivity	
• Sedation		
• Affective blunting		
• Cognitive dulling		
• Social withdrawal		

Table 7.4

Side-Effect Profiles of Some Common Antipsychotics

Compound	Sedative	Anticholinergic	Extrapyramidal
Phenothiazines			
Chlorpromazine	High	High	Low
Thioridazine	High	High	Low
Trifluoperazine	Medium	Medium	High
Fluphenazine	Medium	Medium	High
Thioxanthenes			
Thiothixene	Low	Low	High
Diphenylbutylpiperidines			
Pimozide	Low	Low	High
Butyrophenones			
Haloperidol	Low	Low	High
Dibenzoxapines			
Clozapine	High	High	Low

Diphenhydramine (Benadryl) is primarily antihistaminic, but has significant anticholinergic activity and is more sedating than the other agents noted. Specific treatment guidelines are given below.

Acute Dystonia

Acute dystonia is most common with high-potency agents. It is characterized by sudden cramping and pain, usually involving the head, neck, and back musculature, and can be severe enough to compromise respiration or cause skeletal injury. Oculogyric or opisthotonic crises may occur and, if untreated, can be life-threatening. Subacute cases may present with dysarthria, jaw or tongue cramping, or dysphagia.

The treatment of dystonic reactions is based on rapid introduction of antiparkinsonian agents. The IM or IV injection of diphenhydramine (50 mg) or benztropine (2 mg) is often sufficient for large children and adolescents. Initial doses may be reduced for smaller children, although dystonic reactions are less common in preadolescents.[13] If dystonia fails to resolve within 15 to 20 minutes after the first injection, the dose is

Table 7.5

Acute Management of Adverse Reactions to Antipsychotic Agents

Reaction	Management*
Anticholinergic symptoms	1. Decrease dose 2. Eliminate concurrent anticholinergic drugs 3. Change to higher-potency agent
Extrapyramidal symptoms	1. Decrease dose 2. Add antiparkinsonian agent (e.g., benztropine or biperiden) 3. Change to a lower-potency agent
Acute dystonia	1. Airway management 2. Diphenhydramine 50 mg IM or IV, or benztropine 2 mg IM (may repeat dose every 15–20 min) 3. Lorazepam 1–2 mg IM or IV
Akathisia	1. Decrease dose 2. Antiparkinsonian agents may be tried 3. Propranolol 10–30 mg t.i.d., or clonazepam 0.5–1.0 mg b.i.d.
Neuroleptic malignant syndrome	1. Discontinue neuroleptics 2. Cardiorespiratory support 3. Hydration 4. May use bromocriptine 2.5–10 mg t.i.d., *or* dantrolene 1–3 mg/ky/day, divided 5. Benzodiazepines may alleviate agitation and rigidity
Hyperprolactinemia	1. Reduce or discontinue medication 2. Amantadine 100–300 mg/day, divided, may be effective

*Doses and safety of pharmacologic approaches have not been established for preadolescents.

repeated, followed by either a third dose or augmentation with a rapid-acting benzodiazepine (lorazepam 1 mg IM or IV). Long-term management includes the decrease or discontinuation of the antipsychotic agent, a change to a lower-potency agent, or the addition of regular doses of anti-Parkinsonian agents.

Akathisia

Akathisia is a potential antipsychotic side effect, described as the subjective feeling that one must stay in constant motion. This may or may not be visible to the clinician as restlessness, agitation, or motoric hyperactivity. Decreasing the antipsychotic dose or adding anti-Parkinsonian agents may provide relief.

Unless contraindicated by a history of asthma or insulin-dependent diabetes, the authors recommend trying a low dose of a beta-adrenergic blocking agent, such as propranolol. For young children, it is reasonable to start with a 5-mg test dose, monitoring blood pressure and pulse with each dose change. Subsequent doses should be given on a t.i.d. schedule and titrated to clinical response (20 to 40 mg/day in adolescents and adults).

Trials of benzodiazepines suggest that these agents may equal propranolol in efficacy. However, a reduction of the neuroleptic dose and a trial of propranolol should be tried first, since the long-term use of benzodiazepines may further impair daytime function (see Chapter 10).

Movement Disorders

There are several manifestations of this potentially serious long-term side effect, most involving involuntary, often unconscious, movements of the tongue, face, and neck. Such abnormal involuntary movements may appear after discontinuing antipsychotic therapy (withdrawal dyskinesia) or during chronic therapy (tardive dyskinesia). The latter is rare in patients exposed to neuroleptics for less than six months, but the risk increases with the age of the patient, the length of exposure, and the intensity of exposure (high doses and high potency). Once it emerges, tardive dyskinesia is often a long-term, although not necessarily permanent, problem.

Since there is no proven treatment for neuroleptic-induced dyskinesia, proper management involves thorough pretreatment counseling, minimization of the neuroleptic dose and exposure, and periodic standardized examination for involuntary movements. The Abnormal Involuntary Movement Scale (AIMS) is useful for this purpose (see page 217 in Textbook).[14]

Neuroleptic Malignant Syndrome

This potentially life-threatening adverse reaction to neuroleptics is characterized by fever, lead-pipe muscular rigidity, altered mental status, hyper- or hypotension, tachycardia, diaphoresis, and pallor. Laboratory findings include myoglobinuria and elevations in white blood cell count, hepatic enzymes, and creatinine phosphokinase (CPK usually > 1,000 U/L). The clinical picture may be mistaken for psychosis, catatonia, EPS, infection, or fever of unknown origin.[15]

The risk of NMS appears to be declining, possibly owing to the lower doses of antipsychotics being used today. Recent estimates are as low as 0.15% of patients exposed.[16] However, a number of cases have been reported after brief exposure and in children as young as 11 months of age. The risk of mortality from NMS has likewise decreased, from 25% to approximately 11%.[17]

Treatment usually requires hospitalization, hydration, and cessation of all antidopaminergic and anticholinergic medication. Close monitoring of cardiac and renal status is required to avoid arrhythmias and myonecrotic kidney failure, respectively. Fever may become quite high, requiring cooling. Bromocriptine mesylate, at (adult) doses of 2.5 to 10 mg t.i.d., appears to improve rigidity and mental status, while sodium dantrolene, in four divided doses of 1 to 3 mg/kg/day, may decrease rigidity, tachycardia, and myonecrosis. The agents may be used simultaneously.[15] It should be noted that researchers disagree about whether these pharmacologic treatments of NMS significantly alter the outcome. On the other hand, the incidence of adverse reactions to dantrolene or bromocriptine is low.

The retrial of neuroleptics in a patient who has recovered from NMS remains a controversial issue. Retrial is clearly contraindicated for nonpsychotic patients. Yet, many past victims of NMS require continued treatment for chronic psychosis. In the past, the retrial of antipsychotics was strongly discouraged on the presumption that most patients would suffer recurrent NMS. However, the risk of recurrent NMS is lower than once thought; certainly, it is under 40%, and perhaps much lower.[18,19]

If a retrial is necessary, subsequent antipsychotics should be from a different chemical class, of lower potency, and at a lower equivalent dose than the offending agent. Intensive monitoring for fever and laboratory markers of NMS is necessary. Because of improved prescribing and the rapid decline in NMS cases associated with any antipsychotic, it is unclear whether the incidence of NMS is lower with the newer antipsychotics, such as clozapine and risperidone.

Hyperprolactinemia

Prolonged dopaminergic blockade may produce hyperprolactinemia, which is manifested as galactorrhea (in females or males), amenorrhea, or impotence. The primary treatment is reduction of the dose, although switching to an alternative (usually lower-potency) antipsychotic may also help. Neuroleptic-induced hyperprolactinemia in adults has been successfully treated with dopamine agonists (bromocriptine and amantadine),[20,21] but in our experience, these agents too often exacerbate the underlying psychosis.

Anticholinergic Side Effects

Anticholinergic side effects include blurred vision, constipation, agitation, delirium, and exacerbation of narrow-angle glaucoma. Anticholinergic (usually low-potency) neuroleptics should be avoided when these side effects are of concern, such as in the presence of delirium, other anticholinergic agents (antihistamines and heterocyclic antidepressants), glaucoma, encopresis, or neurologic illness in which level of consciousness must be monitored.

Sudden Death

Several case reports describe sudden, unexplainable demise during treatment with high-potency neuroleptics. In particular, haloperidol and droperidol have been associated with the death of patients while on high, but clinically acceptable, injected doses. The mechanisms and relative risk of this rare reaction are unknown.

Cardiac Effects

Low-potency agents commonly produce postural hypotension and/or syncope, presumably through adrenergic blockade, and may produce quinidine-like effects on cardiac conduction. Cases of heart block and ventricular tachycardia have been reported, especially in overdose. Pimozide and thioridazine are notable for higher incidences of QT prolongation and reports of arrhythmias, even at therapeutic doses.

Agranulocytosis

Reported hematologic effects include leukopenia, thrombocytopenia, and lymphopenia. However, the most serious effect is idiosyncratic agranulocytosis, although it is rare. The risk is highest with clozapine, but exists with most neuroleptics. The manufacturer of clozapine continues to require that each treatment center assess hematologic and cardiac effects weekly in patients receiving clozapine, including weekly complete blood counts (CBCs).

Other adverse effects include sedation and cognitive dulling, increased risk of seizure, hepatic toxicity (especially with chlorpromazine), photosensitivity, and rare ocular pigmentation.

Overdose

Antipsychotic overdose often presents with severe forms of the typical side effects associated with dopamine blockade (Parkinsonian symptoms, dystonia, etc.), particularly with high-potency agents. However, the progression of symptoms depends on the specific agent. With pimozide or thioridazine, cardiac arrhythmias may appear sooner rather than later in the progression of toxic symptoms. More sedating agents may produce CNS and cardiovascular depression, hypotension, and respiratory depression as early signs of toxicity. Anticholinergic delirium may be the initial clinical picture. Hypertension has been reported in childhood overdose of haloperidol.

The treatment of neuroleptic overdose is supportive and symptomatic. Extrapyramidal symptoms and NMS are treated as described above. Cardiac monitoring and respiratory support are needed. There are few reports of death resulting from an overdose of neuroleptics.

Available Preparations

For most applications in children and adolescents, antipsychotics are administered orally. Intramuscular preparations are available for conditions in which rapid absorption is desirable, such as for sedation. Two neuroleptics (haloperidol and fluphenazine) are available in oil-based depot preparations, which are used to extend normal half-lives. Haloperidol decanoate ($t_{1/2}$ = approximately 21 days) is administered monthly, while fluphenazine decanoate ($t_{1/2}$ = 7–10 days) is typically administered twice monthly. These agents are helpful only when the chronic use of high-potency neuroleptics is unavoidable and the extremely long half-lives are needed for compliance—conditions that are rarely encountered in the treatment of children.

Initiating and Maintaining Treatment

It is advisable to complete diagnostic procedures prior to neuroleptic treatment. Baseline CBCs with differential, hepatic enzymes, CPK, blood pressure, ECG, and AIMS examination are needed for later comparison. Antipsychotic agents can also produce abnormalities on the EEG, psychometric testing, and neurologic examination. Baseline measurements of each are preferable, although not always practical. A negative pregnancy test and adequate contraceptive use is recommended for female patients of reproductive age.

Most adverse effects appear within the first two months of starting or increasing medication, but NMS, dyskinesia, and idiosyncratic agranulocytosis may appear at any time during therapy. The laboratory work and AIMS examination should be carried out monthly for the first three months, and every six months thereafter. An ECG should follow any change in dosage of pimozide or thioridazine, in particular. Clozapine requires taking a CBC, blood pressure, and pulse weekly during treatment.

Clinical Practice

Starting and maintenance doses, where established, are listed in Table 7.6. Maintenance doses are determined on an individual basis by starting at the minimal recommended dose

Table 7.6

Approved Age Ranges and Suggested Pediatric Doses for Some Common Antipsychotic Drugs

Compound	Approved Age Range	Recommended Pediatric Doses
Chlorpromazine	>6 months	0.25 mg/kg PO q4–6 h or IM q6–8 h. Max. IM dose is 45 mg/day (<5 yrs) or 75 mg/day (5–12 yrs)
Thioridazine	>2 yrs	0.5 mg/kg/day divided b.i.d. or t.i.d. to max. of 3.0 mg/kg/day for ages 2–12 yrs
Trifluoperazine	>6 yrs	1–15 mg/day given b.i.d. or t.i.d.
Prochlorperazine	>2 yrs	2.5 mg PO b.i.d. or t.i.d. to max. of 20 mg/day (2–5 yrs) or 25 mg/day (6–12 yrs)
Chlorprothixene	>6 yrs	10–25 mg PO t.i.d. or q.i.d. IM route not recommended for under 12 yrs
Pimozide	>2 yrs	1–2 mg/day in divided doses. Max. is lesser of 0.2 mg/kg/day or 10 mg/day
Haloperidol	>3 yrs	0.05–0.15 mg/kg/day divided b.i.d. or t.i.d. for psychosis or 0.05–0.075 for others

Neuroleptic drugs not listed have not been as well studied for children under 12 years of age. Loxapine and clozapine are not recommended for those under 16 years. Pediatric doses have not been established for these agents.

and titrating upward to clinical response or unacceptable side effects. The emergence of EPS may be managed by the addition of antiparkinsonian agents, as described above, but should first prompt a reduction of dose where possible.

Selecting a Specific Agent

In general, clinicians favor low-potency neuroleptics when sedation is desirable (e.g., aggression and agitated psychotic states) and high-potency agents when sedation is undesirable (e.g., Tourette's syndrome and delirium). Beyond this generalization, the specific choice should be based on the patient's symptoms. Recommendations for specific disorders, where available, are given below.

See Table 7.7.

Schizophrenia

Many neuroleptics have been tested for use in childhood schizophrenia and found to be effective for the primary symptoms. However, high-potency agents should be considered first-line therapy when aggression and agitation are absent.[22] As an example, haloperidol may be started at 0.01 to 0.05 mg/kg/day in two or three divided doses for small children, or 0.5 mg b.i.d. for older children and adolescents. The dose is then titrated upward to clinical response or prohibitive side effects. Even in older adolescents, maintenance doses above 15 mg/day seldom add to clinical response.

If dosing is limited by EPS, the clinician should consider adding an anticholinergic compound or switching to an agent of slightly lower potency. If clinical improvement is not observed after two weeks of uninterrupted therapy at maximal doses, consideration should be given to augmentation with lithium or anticonvulsants (Chapters 8 and 9). If compliance becomes a chronic problem, schizophrenia is one of the few acceptable indications for depot antipsychotics in children. Finally, for children with a long history of suboptimal response to classic antipsychotic agents or of intractable EPS, consideration should be given to a newer antipsychotic, clozapine. Clozapine bears higher risks of agranulocytosis and severe sedation, but has a lower incidence of other neuroleptic side effects and may be more efficacious than classic neuroleptics.

Tourette's Disorder

Haloperidol is initiated in the same manner as with schizophrenic children. However, maintenance doses are much lower. The recommended range is 0.05 to 0.075 mg/kg/day or up to 3 mg/day, although doses as high as 10 mg/day are occasionally necessary.[6]

Pimozide is usually titrated to 0.2 mg/kg/day or 10 mg/day, whichever is smaller. Prolongation of QT is evident on ECG at higher doses, and sudden death has occurred at doses above 20 mg/day. Therefore, serial ECGs must be performed during dose titration and periodically during follow-up.

Table 7.7

Relative Potencies of Some Common Antipsychotic Agents

Compound	Trade Name	Clinical Potency*	Dopamine Blockade	Cholinergic Blockade[†]	Dose (mg/day) Range for Adults
Phenothiazines					
Chlorpromazine	Thorazine	1	1.0	330	400–1000
Thioridazine	Mellaril	1	0.72	1,300	200–800
Mesoridazine	Serentil	2	1.0	330	100–400
Trifluoperazine	Stelazine	30	7.2	35	15–40
Fluphenazine	Prolixin	50–100	24	13	2.5–10.0
Perphenazine	Trilafon	10	13	16	16–64
Prochlorperazine	Compazine	7	2.6	43	30–150
Thioxanthenes					
Chlorprothixene	Taractan	1	2.5	—	100–600
Thiothixene	Navane	25	42	8.1	20–60
Indolic compounds					
Molindone	Moban	10	0.16	0.062	50–225
Diphenylbutyl-piperdines					
Pimozide	Orap	≈50	≈5.3	—	1–10
Butyrophenones					
Haloperidol	Haldol	50	4.7	1.0	1–15
Droperidol		—	≈6.2	—	≈8
Dibenzoxapines					
Loxapine	Loxitane	7	0.26	52	60–250
Clozapine	Clozaril	≈1	0.11	2,000	300–900

*Clinical potency and strength of dopamine blockade are expressed as ratios to chlorpromazine.
[†] Strength of cholinergic blockade expressed as ratios to haloperidol.

How to Withdraw Medication

Withdrawal symptoms associated with the abrupt cessation of long-term neuroleptic use include cholinergic rebound (nausea, vomiting, diaphoresis, restlessness, insomnia), withdrawal dyskinesia (including oral dyskinesia, ataxia, or choreiform movements), and psychosis.[23] Thus, withdrawal of the drug should be gradual if treatment has been lengthy.

References

1. American Psychiatric Association. (1994). *Diagnostic and Statistical Manual of Mental Disorders* (4th ed.). Washington, DC: American Psychiatric Association.
2. Burd, L., Kerbeshian, J. (1987). A North Dakota prevalence study of schizophrenia presenting in childhood. *J Am Acad Child Adolesc Psychiatry, 26,* 347–350.
3. Kotsopoulos, S., Kanigsberg, J., Cote, A., Fiedorowicz, C. (1987). Hallucinatory experiences in nonpsychotic children. *J Am Acad Child Adolesc Psychiatry, 26,* 375–380.
4. May, P.R.A., Tuma, H., Yale, C., et al. (1976). Schizophrenia—A follow-up study of results of treatment: II. Hospital stay over two to five years. *Arch Gen Psychiatry, 33,* 481–486.
5. Shapiro, A.K., Shapiro, E., Fulop, G. (1987). Pimozide treatment of tic and Tourette disorders. *Pediatrics, 79,* 1032–1039.
6. Erenberg, G. (1988). Pharmacologic therapy of tics in childhood. *Pediatr Ann, 17,* 395–404.
7. Gittelman-Klein, R., Klein, D.F., Katz, S., et al. (1976). Comparative effects of methylphenidate and thioridazine in hyperactive children. I. Clinical results. *Arch Gen Psychiatry, 33,* 1217–1231.
8. Weizman, A., Weitz, R., Szekely, G.A., et al. (1984). Combination of neuroleptic and stimulant treatment in attention deficit disorder with hyperactivity. *J Am Acad Child Psychiatry, 23,* 295–298.
9. Sprague, R.L., Barnes, K.R., Werry, J.S. (1970). Methylphenidate and thioridazine: Learning, reaction time, activity and classroom behavior in disturbed children. *Am J Orthopsychiatry, 40,* 615–628.
10. Farber, J.M. (1987). Psychopharmacology of self-injurious behavior in the mentally retarded. *J Am Acad Child Adolesc Psychiatry, 26,* 296–302.
11. Stewart, J.T., Myers, W.C., Burket, R.C., Lyles, W.B. (1990). A review of the pharmacology of aggression in children and adolescents. *J Am Acad Child Adolesc Psychiatry, 29,* 269–277.
12. Campbell, M., Small, A.M., Green, W.H., et al. (1984). Behavioral efficacy of haloperidol and lithium carbonate: A comparison in

hospitalized aggressive children with conduct disorder. *Arch Gen Psychiatry, 41,* 650–656.

13. Campbell, M. (1985). Schizophrenic disorders and pervasive developmental disorders/infantile autism. In J.M. Wiener (Ed.), *Diagnosis and Psychopharmacology of Childhood and Adolescent Disorders* (pp. 114–150). New York: Wiley.

14. National Institute of Mental Health. (1985). AIMS (Abnormal Involuntary Movement Scale). *Psychopharmacol Bull, 21,* 1077–1080.

15. Harpe, C., Stoudemire, A. (1987). Etiology and treatment of neuroleptic malignant syndrome. *Med Toxicol, 2,* 166–176.

16. Keck, P.E., Jr., Pope, H.G., Jr., McElroy, S.L. (1991). Declining frequency of neuroleptic malignant syndrome in a hospital population. *Am J Psychiatry, 148,* 880–882.

17. Shalev, A., Hermesh, H., Munitz, H. (1989). Mortality from neuroleptic malignant syndrome. *J Clin Psychiatry, 50,* 18–25.

18. Addonizio, G., Susman, V.L., Roth, S.D. (1987). Neuroleptic malignant syndrome: Review and analysis of 115 cases. *Biol Psychiatry, 22,* 1004–1020.

19. Pelonero, A.L., Levenson, J.L., Silvermann, J.J. (1985). Neuroleptic therapy following neuroleptic malignant syndrome. *Psychosomatics, 26,* 946–948.

20. Cohn, J.B., Brust, J., DiSerio, F., Singer, J. (1985). Effect of bromocriptine mesylate on induced hyperprolactinemia in stabilized psychiatric outpatients undergoing neuroleptic treatment. *Neuropsychobiology, 13,* 173–179.

21. Correa, N., Opler, L.A., Kay, S.R., Birmaher, B. (1987). Amantadine in the treatment of neuroendocrine side effects of neuroleptics. *J Clin Psychopharmacol, 7,* 91–95.

22. Realmuto, G.M., Erickson, W.D., Yellin, A.M., et al. Clinical comparison of thiothixene and thioridazine in schizophrenic adolescents. *Am J Psychiatry, 141,* 440–442.

23. Gardos, G., Cole, J.O., Tarsy, D. (1978). Withdrawal syndromes associated with antipsychotic drugs. *Am J Psychiatry, 135,* 1321–1324.

C h a p t e r   8

Lithium

Lithium is the drug of choice for the treatment of adults with bipolar disorder.[1] While there are no extensive, placebo-controlled, double-blind studies assessing lithium's efficacy in treating bipolar disorder in children and adolescents, open-label studies have revealed that it can be helpful in this population.[2] Lithium's only FDA-established indication, however, is for the acute and maintenance treatment of bipolar disorders in patients at least 12 years old.

Chemical Properties

See Table 8.1.

Lithium carbonate (Li_2CO_3) is a very soluble cation salt that is rapidly absorbed after oral administration. A citrate form of lithium is also available as a syrup that contains 8 mEq lithium/5 ml. Peak blood levels are achieved within approximately two hours for standard preparations of lithium, while peak levels for the sustained-release form are generally achieved within four and one-half hours.[1] It is excreted predominantly by the kidney, with approximately 80% being reabsorbed in the proximal renal tubules.

In adults, the elimination half-life of lithium is approximately 24 hours, and over 60% of an acute dose is excreted within 12 hours. Children generally have a shorter elimination half-life of lithium, and its steady-state levels are reached sooner in children than in adults.

Table 8.1

Pharmacokinetic Properties of Lithium

Absorption	Peak Serum Levels (Hours)	Serum Half-Life (Hours)	Principal Route of Excretion
Gastrointestinal	2–4	20–24	Renal

Table 8.2

Indications for Lithium in Child and Adolescent Psychiatry

FDA Established:
- Bipolar disorder—acute mania in patients >12 years
- Prophylaxis for bipolar disorder in patients >12 years

Possible Indications:
- Bipolar disorder—acute mania in children <12 years
- Bipolar disorder—acute depression
- Unipolar depression
- Augmentation of tricyclic-refractory depression
- Prophylaxis for unipolar depression
- Cyclothymia
- Psychosis
- Aggression and violent behavior
- ADHD
- Alcohol abuse/dependence
- Bulimia
- Personality disorders
- Functional encopresis

Indications

See Table 8.2.

Bipolar Disorder

Acute Mania

In clinical practice, the guidelines that apply to lithium's use in adults also are commonly used for younger patients,[3] although children and adolescents are able to tolerate higher oral doses.[4]

As in adults, the addition of a neuroleptic may be required for early behavioral control. However, caution and restraint should be exercised in adding a neuroleptic because of adverse neurologic reactions. In bipolar disorder, it generally takes longer to produce a positive response to lithium therapy, but when successful, the response may be more complete.

Acute Depression
Lithium is not effective as often as antidepressants are (see Chapter 4) in the treatment of acute depressive episodes in adult patients with bipolar disorder.[5] Still, most experts advise maximizing the lithium dose for depressive symptoms of bipolar disorder before adding antidepressants. In adults, it is usual to add an antidepressant to lithium for bipolar disorder, depressed type. There are no data on children and adolescents. However, this has to be assessed within the context that antidepressants have not been established as effective in child and adolescent depression (see Chapter 4). One should check thyroid function when a child or adolescent on lithium becomes depressed, since lithium can cause hypothyroidism, sometimes resulting in decreased energy levels and other depressive signs and symptoms.

Prophylaxis of Bipolar Disorder
In adults, lithium is indicated for the prophylactic treatment of bipolar disorder.[6] It appears to be less effective in decreasing depressive recurrences than manic recurrences. There are no prophylactic data on children and adolescents. If a child or adolescent has responded well to lithium, it is advisable to keep him or her on a maintenance dose for a minimum of six to nine months.

Unipolar Depression

Lithium is not believed to be as effective as antidepressants in the treatment of unipolar depression in adults.[7] There are no data on children and adolescents on the use of lithium alone in the treatment of an acute unipolar depression.

Interest is being generated in using lithium to augment the effects of antidepressants, such as TCAs and SSRIs, to treat refractory depression in children and adolescents, and this is based on augmentation studies in adults.[8] Ryan et al.[8] reported that 6 of 14 children and adolescents had a good response on lithium augmentation of a TCA. All tolerated the combination well without toxicity. The duration of lithium augmentation required to produce a significant clinical response was longer than that reported in the adult literature.[8]

Prophylaxis for Unipolar Depression
In contrast to bipolar prophylaxis where lithium is considered to be the drug of choice, most psychiatrists do not use lithium as a first-line agent for the prophylaxis of unipolar depression in adults. There are no data on children and adolescents.

Cyclothymia

Cyclothymia is characterized by periods of hypomania alternating with periods of depression not severe enough to meet the criteria for a major depressive episode or mania. Since cyclothymic patients often have a family history of mood disorders and may look similar to rapid-cycling bipolar disorder patients, a lithium trial is probably worthwhile as long as there are no confounding factors affecting the diagnosis.

Psychosis

Limited experience with children and adolescents suggests that lithium may exert a beneficial effect on psychoses with manic features.[2] If lithium alone is not completely effective, one may add either carbamazepine or valproic acid. Antipsychotics should be reserved for either initial short-term use until behavior control is established or as a last resort for long-term therapy.

In summary, when mood symptoms are observed during a psychotic process, lithium therapy should be considered. In fact, lithium's mood-stabilizing properties may be particularly beneficial in psychotic patients prone to disconcerting shifts in their moods.

Severe Aggression and Explosive Behavior

Observations of adults in several noncontrolled studies have shown that lithium is effective in decreasing episodic and explosive behavior in patients with a variety of diagnostic conditions, including antisocial personality disorder. One major controlled study[9] of children and adolescents showed that lithium is more effective than placebo in treating conduct disorder and undersocialized aggression. In all of these instances, lithium was noted to be especially helpful in decreasing explosive behavior. In the controlled study with a haloperidol comparison group, it was shown to cause fewer and less toxic side effects than haloperidol. These observations also have been made with regard to children with behavior disorders with a variety of concomitant neurologic conditions, including mental retardation with and without encopresis. In one of the studies,[10] the mean serum lithium levels were 0.68 mEq/L, and thus within the acceptable therapeutic range.

Attention-Deficit/Hyperactivity Disorder
It is only when more standard treatments of ADHD are unsuccessful that alternative medications, such as lithium, carbamazepine, or antipsychotics, are considered.

Contraindications
See Table 8.3.

Pregnancy
Lithium use, particularly in the first trimester of pregnancy, significantly increases the risk of cardiac deformities and malformations.

Table 8.3

Contraindications to Lithium Use in Child and Adolescent Psychiatry

Absolute:
• Allergic drug reaction (rare)
Relative:
• Pregnancy
• Renal disease
• Cardiovascular disease
• Thyroid disease
• Severe dehydration/sodium depletion

Renal disease

Lithium is relatively contraindicated for children and adolescents with renal disease as it is primarily excreted by the kidneys.

Cardiovascular Disease

Lithium is relatively contraindicated for children and adolescents with cardiovascular disease as it has been associated with atrioventricular block and other cardiovascular side effects. Its use in such patients can significantly raise the likelihood that lithium toxicity will develop.[11]

Thyroid Disease

Thyroid disease is no longer felt to be an absolute contraindication to lithium's use. Carefully monitoring thyroid function and using supplemental thyroxine (Synthroid) when necessary. It is appropriate to adjust the lithium dose to its lowest level of effectiveness.

Severe Dehydration/Sodium Depletion

Severe dehydration and sodium depletion are relative contraindications to lithium's use for children and adolescents because of the very high risk of toxicity.

Patients on Thiazides

Lithium is not contraindicated for patients taking thiazides, although an alternative dosing strategy is necessary for these patients.

Side Effects

See Table 8.4.

Gastrointestinal Discomfort

Signs and symptoms of GI discomfort include nausea, vomiting, loose stools, abdominal discomfort, and irritation and feelings of malaise. These effects are usually short-lived and may be related to peak plasma lithium levels. Having the patient take lithium with meals may help ameliorate GI symptoms. Starting with a low dose and increasing the dose gradually so that the patient becomes tolerant to the medication may be helpful. Sustained-release lithium preparations (e.g., Lithobid) may be

Table 8.4

Side Effects of Lithium

Common:
- GI (nausea/vomiting, diarrhea)
- Tremor
- Leukocytosis
- Malaise

Uncommon:
- Renal (polydipsia/polyuria)
- Ocular irritation/stomatitis
- Hypothyroidism/nontoxic goiter
- Dermatologic
- Cardiovascular
- Weight gain/edema
- NMS/encephalopathic syndrome
- Diabetes
- Hair loss
- Growth and development

---

tolerated better. Cessation of lithium therapy should be considered if its use results in significant electrolyte and volume depletion via emesis and/or diarrhea.

Tremor

A fine tremor is often seen early during lithium treatment and is in contrast to the gross tremor seen with lithium toxicity.

Renal Dysfunction

Polyuria and polydipsia may occur at any time during lithium therapy because of its direct effect on the kidneys,[6] and can result in a nephrogenic diabetes insipidus–like syndrome. This side effect may necessitate decreasing the dose, discontinuing the lithium, or, more rarely, treating the condition with chlorothiazide. Patients who suffer from severe polyuria secondary to lithium have been reported to excrete several liters of urine per day. It is, therefore, essential that kidney function be monitored since lithium has been rarely reported to result in a decreased glomerular filtration rate as a result of glomerular sclerosis and tubular atrophy.

Hypothyroidism/Nontoxic Goiter

Lithium can produce hypothyroidism and nontoxic goiter.[12] Decreased circulating thyroid hormones T_3 and T_4 and elevated tythroid-simulating hormone (TSH) may result. Hyperthyroidism has been reported rarely.

Dermatologic Effects

Dermatologic side effects include an increase in acne vulgaris and maculopapular eruptions or exacerbation and/or aggravation of psoriasis.

Leukocytosis

Lithium not infrequently causes a clinically insignificant increase in the white blood cell count of between 10,000 and 15,000 cells/mm^3, with increased polymorphonuclear leukocytes, lymphocytopenia, and platelet count.[13] This does not appear to have any untoward significance.

Malaise and Fatigue

Malaise and fatigue are not uncommonly seen in patients receiving lithium. Children and adolescents may complain of feeling sluggish, tired, and uncomfortable, but this does not always imply toxicity. Sometimes these feelings disappear with time as the child adjusts to the medication, or they may necessitate decreasing the dose.

Neuroleptic Malignant Syndrome

The syndrome has been seen in patients treated with a combination of lithium and antipsychotic medications. In a few such patients, a full-blown encephalopathic syndrome has developed, which is characterized by weakness, lethargy, fever, confusion, extrapyramidal side effects, increased white blood cell count, increased blood urea nitrogen (BUN), increased serum enzymes, and increased fasting blood sugar. This usually occurs at toxic plasma lithium levels. If such symptoms are seen, discontinuing the medication is necessary (see Chapter 7).

Overdose/Toxicity

Lithium toxicity is very closely related to serum lithium levels, and may be seen at doses close to therapeutic levels. The clinician must monitor the patient closely to determine any condition that can alter the sodium balance, such as dehydration or a change in diet. It is important that the patient and family be advised that the child or adolescent on lithium should get sufficient amounts of table salt and liquids.

Mild intoxication can manifest as subtle symptoms, such as GI distress or dizziness. In these cases, the lithium should be withheld until the level returns to the therapeutic range.[5] It is important to search for the cause of the increased level (noncompliance, accidental overingestion, etc.). If no obvious cause for the increased level and toxicity is found, a renal workup is indicated, which should include a urinalysis, electrolytes, BUN and creatinine, creatinine clearance, urinary sodium, and 24-hour protein. Moderate or severe lithium toxicity requires the patient to be admitted to the hospital so that sodium can be administered while frequent monitoring of lithium levels is carried out.[5]

Acute Lithium Intoxication

See Table 8.5.

Lithium levels above 3 mmol/L can be life-threatening and represent a medical emergency.[5] The reversibility of lithium intoxication is directly related to the serum level of lithium and the length of time it remains elevated. It is important that

Table 8.5

Acute Lithium Intoxication Treatment

- There is no specific antidote to lithium poisoning
- The principles of treatment are similar to those for barbiturate overdose
- Monitor airway, breathing, and circulation
- Obtain toxicologic screen for other drugs
- Gastric lavage
- Correct fluid/electrolyte imbalance promptly
- Levels <3 mmol/L—less severe poisoning

Institute IV Therapy with Normal Saline at 150–200 ml/Hour as Long as the Patient is Producing Adequate Urine

- At levels >3 mmol/L—evidence of severe toxicity (often minimal urine output and/or renal failure). Hemodialysis is necessary
- Urea, mannitol, and aminophylline can increase lithium excretion
- Goal: reduce lithium level to <1 mmol/L at six hours after dialysis

immediate measures be taken to reduce the toxic level. Severe symptoms can arise suddenly and without warning, resulting in the death of the patient. Signs of serious lithium intoxication include ataxia, dysarthria, gross tremor, delirium, hallucinations, seizure, coma, renal failure, diarrhea, and neuromuscular irritability or flaccidity.[5] Patients who survive severe lithium toxicity may suffer permanent impairment of their memory, gait, and other functions.

There is no specific antidote to lithium poisoning. The clinician should obtain a toxicologic screen to see if the patient has taken any other drugs. Treatment is very similar to that for barbiturate overdoses. Gastric lavage should be undertaken in acute overdose patients.[5] Lithium levels are often quite high in gastric secretions, so gastric aspiration is very important.[5] It is also essential that correction of the fluid and electrolyte imbalance be initiated promptly. When lithium levels are less than 3 mmol/L and the signs of intoxication are mild, this fluid and electrolyte imbalance can be corrected by administering IV normal saline at rates of 150 to 200 ml/hour as long as the patient is producing adequate urine.[5] At lithium levels greater than 3 mmol/L and with evidence of severe toxicity (i.e., if there is minimal urine output and/or renal failure), dialysis is necessary. Hemodialysis is the preferred treatment, as it rapidly removes lithium ions from the toxic patient. Urea, mannitol, and aminophylline are capable of significantly increasing the excretion of lithium. It is very important to monitor lithium levels frequently during dialysis, as lithium will reequilibrate from the tissues after hemodialysis treatment.[5] Targeted lithium levels are 1 mmol/L or less six hours after dialysis. When such levels are reached, the dialysis can be stopped. As with any overdose, it is also important to monitor the patient's airway, breathing, and circulation.

Initiating and Maintaining Treatment

See Table 8.6.

Before treatment with lithium is begun in children and adolescents, a premedication workup is required that is similar to that performed on adults. Children and adolescents must have a complete history taken and physical examination

Table 8.6

Lithium Drug Interactions

Increase Serum Lithium Levels:

- Antibiotics
- Carbamazepine
- Diuretics
- Nonsteroidal anti-inflammatory agents

Decrease Serum Lithium Levels:

- Acetazolamide
- Caffeine
- Osmotic diuretics
- Theophylline

Interact with Lithium to Produce Sedation and/or Confusional States:

- Alcohol
- Antihypertensives
- Antipsychotics (especially haloperidol)

---

performed by their primary medical physician. Laboratory assessment includes a pregnancy test on every female patient, because lithium crosses the placenta and is associated with an increased risk of congenital heart disease in infants born to mothers using lithium during pregnancy. The period of greatest risk appears to be the first trimester. The most common cardiac malformation is Ebstein's anomaly, but other cardiac disturbances can occur in these infants, and there is also an increased risk for cyanosis, hypotonia, and lethargy.

It is important to assess all children and adolescents for evidence of kidney and thyroid disease before lithium is started, in order to ascertain the patient's baseline function. In healthy patients, this merely requires checking a urinalysis for BUN and creatinine.[14] If a renal anomaly is noted prior to initiating lithium therapy, it is probably best to avoid lithium and to try an alternative medication, such as carbamazepine. Laboratory tests to be checked include a urinalysis (paying particular attention to specific gravity), BUN and creatinine, creatinine clearance, 24-hour urine protein, and urinary sodium. If any anomaly is noted, such as the child going to the bathroom more frequently than usual, drinking more fluids than usual, or complaining of increased thirst, the parents should be instructed to call the psychiatrist immediately, and to withhold the lithium until they speak with the doctor and/or have the child assessed.

Children and adolescents treated with lithium should have a CBC with differential and platelet count, since lithium is known to cause a leukocytosis with neutrophilia, lymphocytopenia, and increased platelet counts in some patients.[13] The leukocytosis is benign, and can often be distinguished from leukocytosis caused by true infection, since during lithium therapy the neutrophils are more mature in form, whereas infection affects the younger forms of neutrophils. Lithium does not have to be discontinued when a leukocytosis develops.

Children who have conduct disorders have been observed to have increased EEG abnormalities, including focal and paroxysmal changes, while on lithium, as compared with EEGs done prior to treatment.[15] These EEG anomalies do not, however, correlate with lithium toxicity. We do not recommend routine EEGs for children with conduct disorders treated with lithium unless focal neurologic abnormalities are present.

Clinical Practice

Dosage and Administration
See Table 8.7.

For children older than 12 years of age, lithium is started at a low dose and gradually increased, with a repeated monitoring of lithium level.

Starting with an initial dose of 150 to 300 mg of lithium carbonate per day and gradually increasing the dose in 150- to 300-mg increments every five to seven days is advisable. Many of the averse side effects of lithium that occur early during treatment—including GI irritation, such as nausea/vomiting and diarrhea; dizziness and confusion; muscle aches; weakness; polyuria and polydipsia; and hand tremor—take place when the dose of lithium is increased too rapidly, so that serum lithium levels rise too quickly for the body to adjust to them. It will also

Table 8.7

Dosage and Administration of Lithium for Children and Adolescents

Children <12 Years:	Children >12 Years:
Not FDA approved	FDA approved (see Indications, Table 8.2)
Guidelines from Weller and Colleagues*:	Start with dose 150–300 mg/day. Check serum levels five days after dose. Increase gradually by 150–300 mg every five to seven days. For acute mania, doses of 1,800 mg/day (serum level 1–1.5 mEq/L) usually required. For long-term maintenance, doses of 900–1,200 mg/day are usually required, yielding serum levels of 0.6–1.2 mEq/L.
<25 kg, initial dose on t.i.d. schedule: 150/150/300 25–40 kg—300/300/300 40–50 kg—300/300/600 50–60 kg—600/300/600	
• Targeted therapeutic serum levels 0.6–1.2 mEq/L.	
• Should not exceed serum level of 1.4 mEq/L.	
• Increase dose gradually, monitoring efficacy versus toxicity.	
• Keep on specific dose five to seven days.	
• Draw lithium levels 12 hours after giving medication.	

*Adapted from Weller, E.B., Weller, R.A., Fristad, M.A. (1986). Lithium dosage guide for prepubertal children. *J Am Acad Child Psychiatry, 25*, 92–95.

help if the lithium is taken after eating. If the symptoms persist, it might be helpful to switch to enteric-coated lithium, such as Lithobid tablets, or to another slow-release form, such as Eskalith CR, which can be administered twice a day.

Lithium blood levels should be checked five days after the dose is increased, on a later day for slow-release preparations. Because of their increased renal clearance, it is not uncommon for children and adolescents to require higher doses of lithium than adults—1,800 mg/day or more.[16,17] This dosage often results in lithium levels of 1 to 1.5 mEq/L, which may be necessary to control an acute mania. However, the dosage must be adjusted when the manic phase abates (i.e., the dose lowered). Long-term maintenance therapy usually involves the administration of 900 to 1,200 mg of lithium carbonate daily in three or four divided doses, which usually produce levels of 0.6 to 1.2 mEq/L.

References

1. Jefferson, J.W., Greist, J.H., Ackerman, D.L. (1987). *Lithium Encyclopedia for Clinical Practice*. Washington, DC: American Psychiatric Press.
2. Varanka, T.M., Weller, R.A., Weller, E.B., Fristad, M.A. (1988). Lithium treatment of manic episodes with psychotic features in prepubertal children. *Am J Psychiatry*, *145*, 1557–1559.
3. Delong, G.R., Aldershof, A.L. (1987). Long-term experience with lithium treatment in childhood: Correlation with clinical diagnosis. *J Am Acad Child Adolesc Psychiatry*, *26*, 389–394.
4. Ryan, N.D., Puig-Antich, J. (1987). Pharmacological treatment of adolescent psychiatric disorders. *J Adolesc Health Care*, *8*, 137–142.
5. Arana, G.W., Hyman, S.E. (1991). *Handbook of Psychiatric Drug Therapy* (2nd ed.) (pp. 162–170). Boston: Little Brown.
6. Lapierre, Y.D., Raval, K.J. (1989). Pharmacotherapy of affective disorders in children and adolescents. *Psychiat Clin North Am*, *12*, 4.
7. Mendels, J., Ramsey, A., Dyson, W.L., Frazer, A. (1979). Lithium as an antidepressant. *Arch Gen Psychiatry*, *36*, 845.
8. Ryan, N.D., Meyer, V., Dachille, S., et al. (1988). Lithium antidepressant augmentation in TCA-refractory depression. *J Am Acad Child Adolesc Psychiatry*, *27*, 371–376.
9. Campbell, M., Small, A.M., Green, W.H., et al. (1984). Behavioral efficacy of haloperidol and lithium carbonate—comparison in hospitalized aggressive children with conduct disorder. *Arch Gen Psychiatry*, *41*, 650–656.
10. Vetro, A., Szentistvangi, I., Pallag, L., et al. (1985). Therapeutic experience with lithium in childhood aggressivity. *Pharmacopsychiatry*, *14*, 121–127.
11. Jefferson, J.W., Greist, J.H. (1991). Lithium therapy. In H.I. Kaplan, B.J. Sadock (Eds.), *Comprehensive Textbook of Psychiatry* (5th ed.) (p. 1661). Baltimore: Williams & Wilkins.
12. Herskowitz, J. (1987). Developmental neurotoxicology. In C. Popper (Ed.), *Psychiatric Pharmacoscience of Children and Adolescents* (pp. 81–123). Washington, DC: American Psychiatric Press.
13. Reisberg, B., Gershon, S. (1979). Side effects associated with lithium therapy. *Arch Gen Psychiatry*, *36*, 879–887.
14. Rosse, R.B., Geise, A.A., Deutsch, S.I., Morihisa, J.M. (1989). *Laboratory Diagnostic Testing in Psychiatry*. Washington, DC: American Psychiatric Press.
15. Bennett, W.G., Korein, J., Kalmyn, M., et al. (1983). Electroencephalogram and treatment of hospitalized aggressive

children with haloperidol or lithium. *Biol Psychiatry*, *12*, 1427–1440.

16. Jefferson, J.W. (1982). The use of lithium in childhood and adolescence: An overview. *J Clin Psychiatry*, *43*, 174–177.
17. Weller, E.B., Weller, R.A., Fristad, M.A. (1986). Lithium dosage guide for prepubertal children. *J Am Acad Child Psychiatry*, *25*, 92–95.

C h a p t e r   9

Anticonvulsants

Anticonvulsants have established efficacy in the treatment of psychiatric disorders in adults. Carbamazepine and valproic acid have become first-line agents in the treatment of mood disorders. Little data are available on their role in child and adolescent psychiatry.

See Table 9.1.

Carbamazepine has linear kinetics, so a dose increase will result in a predicted increase in serum blood levels.[1]

Valproic acid has a much longer duration of action since its effects on the brain last longer than the drug remains in the blood, making monitoring of serum levels less helpful in predicting responsiveness to the medication.

Phenytoin follows zero-order kinetics. Therefore, there is a nonlinear relationship between dose and serum level.

Carbamazepine, valproic acid, and phenytoin are highly protein bound (over 90%). When protein binding capacity is altered, marked changes occur in the free fractions of these agents, the fractions that can penetrate the blood–brain barrier and enter the brain.

Indications

See Table 9.2.

Bipolar Disorder
Carbamazepine has demonstrated efficacy in adults with bipolar disorder and is often used in patients who do not

Table 9.1

Pharmacokinetic Properties of Anticonvulsants

Drug	Elimination	Protein Binding (%)	Half-Life (hours)	Desired Serum Level (μg/ml)
Carbamazepine	Hepatic	40–90	12	8–12
Valproic acid	Renal	95	8–20	50–100
Phenytoin	Hepatic	90	10–34	10–20
Phenobarbital	Hepatic	50	46–136	20–40
Primidone	Hepatic	80	3–19	8–12
Ethosuximide	Hepatic	0	50–70	80–100

Table 9.2

Indications for Anticonvulsants

Established:
- Bipolar disorder in adults
- Chronic pain/pain associated with nerve injury

Possible:
- Bipolar disorder in children and adolescents
- Major depression
- Intermittent explosive disorder
- ADHD
- Conduct disorders
- Psychotic disorders as adjunct
- Functional enuresis
- Sleep terror disorder

adequately respond to lithium.[2] It has both antimanic and antidepressive effects,[3] and may be used alone or as an adjunct to lithium.[4] There are no data on children.

The antimanic properties of valproic acid have not been definitely established, but many think it to be as effective as, or perhaps more effective than, carbamazepine for bipolar disorder. There are no data in children.

Major Depressive Disorder

Carbamazepine is weaker and less rapid as an antidepressant than as an antimanic agent and was found to improve depression in only a minority of patients.[4,5] It is, therefore, a treatment of last resort for patients with major depression. There are some open clinical data that suggest this agent may be useful for dysphoric children, but more research is needed.

Valproic acid is not believed to be effective in the treatment of pure unipolar major depressive disorder.

Alcohol Withdrawal

In one controlled, randomized double-blind study of 86 male adults with severe alcohol withdrawal, carbamazepine 800 mg/day was found to be as effective as oxazepam 120 mg/day in the treatment of these patients.[6] There have been other open trials in which carbamazepine successfully detoxified patients from benzodiazepines, including diazepam and alprazolam, which are often quite difficult to taper in addicted patients. There are no data on children and adolescents. Carbamazepine, which is not addictive, may offer certain advantages for those children and adolescents who are having some difficulty while they are being detoxified, even if they are not actually suffering a severe, life-threatening withdrawal reaction.[7]

The other anticonvulsants are believed to have very limited use in the treatment of alcohol withdrawal.

Intermittent Explosive Disorder

In open clinical trials, many children with intermittent explosive disorder, particularly those who also have EEG abnormalities, have shown improvement while on carbamazepine.[8] Similar results have been claimed for valproic acid but the number of subjects studied with this agent is much smaller. While phenytoin has also been reported to be of use for this disorder, it is rarely used today because of its variable absorption and high incidence of side effects, thus making carbamazepine and valproic acid the preferred agents.

Chronic Pain

In adults, carbamazepine is the treatment of choice for chronic pain due to trigeminal neuralgia.[9] It is also helpful for the treatment of pain associated with specific nerve damage or injury, neuropathies secondary to diabetes, multiple sclerosis, herpes, and injury or trauma to peripheral neurons.

Phenytoin has also been found to be effective in the treatment of trigeminal neuralgia and other neuropathies.[9]

There are no data on the use of these agents for pain syndromes in children and adolescents.

Attention-Deficit/Hyperactivity Disorder

A large open series has suggested the efficacy of carbamazepine for ADHD in nonepileptic children and adolescents.[10] However, there are no data comparing the treatment with stimulants or other agents with proven efficacy in this disorder. Anecdotal reports suggest that valproic acid may also be useful for this disorder. Clonazepam should be avoided because of the hazard of paradoxical behavioral rebound. (See Chapter 10).

Conduct Disorders in Children and Adolescents

In a single double-blind, placebo-controlled crossover trial of 20 children and adolescents with conduct disorder, carbamazepine was found to be superior to placebo, and higher serum levels (8 to 12 μg/ml) were associated with decreased problem behavior.[11] Phenobarbital should not be used because of the paradoxical worsening of behavior. There are no current data on treatment with valproic acid, phenytoin, or the other anticonvulsants.

Psychosis

Carbamazepine and valproic acid may be helpful as an adjunct to antipsychotic medication in adults with psychosis and affective symptomatology (i.e., schizoaffective disorder).

Functional Enuresis

Carbamazepine decreased enuresis in eight of nine children who had severe behavioral disorders. However, its use for the routine treatment of enuresis cannot be advised because of the lack of data on this usage and the availability of other treatments.

Sleep Terror Disorder

In one study, carbamazepine was found to be helpful in night terrors and other sleep disorders; however, this would not normally be the first- or second-line treatment of these disorders in children.

See Tables 9.3 and 9.4.

Table 9.3

Contraindications to Specific Anticonvulsants

Carbamazepine

Absolute:
- Known hypersensitivity to carbamazepine or TCAs
- History of bone marrow depression
- On MAOI within past two weeks
- Pregnancy

Relative:
- Liver disease
- Kidney disease

Valproic Acid

Absolute:
- Known sensitivity to valproic acid or related drug
- History of bone marrow depression
- Pregnancy
- Age less than 3 years (because of increased risk for liver toxicity)
- Taking clonazepam

Relative:
- Liver disease
- Kidney disease

Phenytoin

Absolute:
- Known hypersensitivity to phenytoin or related drug
- Pregnancy

Relative:
- Alcohol use/dependence
- Cardiac disorders
- Diabetes
- Liver disease
- Renal disease

Table 9.4

Side Effects of Carbamazepine

Common:
- Diplopia (often remits spontaneously or with dosage reduction)
- Drowsiness (usually transient, seen at the beginning of therapy or when dose is increased too rapidly)
- Incoordination

(Continued)

Table 9.4

(Continued)

- Nystagmus
- Nausea
- Leukopenia
- Skin rashes (because of the occasional occurrence of Stevens-Johnson syndrome or systemic lupus erythematosus–like syndrome, discontinuation of mediation and medical consultation may be advised)

Uncommon:

- Agranulocytosis and aplastic anemia
- Hyponatremia and water intoxication (may be more likely when used in conjunction with lithium treatment)
- Liver toxicity
- Neurotoxicity
- Mania
- Exacerbation/precipitation of behavior problems
- Hypocalcemia

References

1. Trimble, M.R. (1990). Anticonvulsants in children and adolescents. *J Child Adolesc Psychopharmacol, 1*, 2.
2. Stuppaeck, C., Barnas, C., Miller, C., et al. (1990). Carbamazepine in the prophylaxis of mood disorders. *J Clin Psychopharmacol, 10*, 39–42.
3. Post, R.M. (1987). Mechanisms of action of carbamazepine and related anticonvulsants in affective illness. In H.Y. Meltzer (Ed.), *Psychopharmacology: The Third Generation of Progress* (pp. 567–576). New York: Raven Press.
4. Schaffer, C.B., Mungas, D., Rockwell, E. (1985). Successful treatment of psychotic depression with carbamazepine. *J Clin Psychopharmacol, 5*, 233.
5. Okuma, T., Ianagu, K., Otsuki, S., et al. (1981). A preliminary double-blind study on the efficacy of carbamazepine in prophylaxis of manic-depressive illness. *Psychopharmacology, 73*, 95–96.
6. Malcolm, R., Ballenger, J.C., Sturgis, E.T., Anton, R. (1989). Double-blind controlled trial comparing carbamazepine to oxazepam treatment of alcohol withdrawal. *Am J Psychiatry, 146*, 617.
7. Ries, R.K., Roy-Byrne, P.P., Ward, N.G., et al. (1989). Carbamazepine treatment for benzodiazepine withdrawal. *Am J Psychiatry, 145*, 536.

8. Kuhn-Gebhardt, V. (1976). Behavioral disorders in non-epileptic children and their treatment with carbamazepine. In W. Birkmayer (Ed.), *Epileptic Seizures—Behavior—Pain* (pp. 264–267). Bern: Hans Huber.
9. Arana, G.W., Hyman, S.E. (1991). *Handbook of Psychiatric Drug Therapy* (2nd ed.). Boston: Little Brown.
10. Remschmidt, H. (1976). The psychotropic effect of carbamazepine in non-epileptic patients, with particular reference to problems posed by clinical studies in children with behavioral disorders. In W. Birkmayer (Ed.), *Epileptic Seizures—Behavior—Pain*. Bern: Hans Huber.
11. Groh, C. (1976). The psychotropic effect of Tegretol in non-epileptic children with particular reference to the drug's indications. In W. Birkmayer (Ed.), *Epileptic Seizures—Behavior—Pain* (pp. 259–263). Bern: Hans Huber.

Anxiolytics and Sedatives

Anxiolytic and sedative agents remain among the most frequently prescribed drugs in medicine, although they have very few recommended applications in child psychiatry. Agents of interest today include benzodiazepines, antihistamines, and azapirones (buspirone). Barbiturates were widely prescribed in the past for a variety of conditions, but have no modern indication for child and adolescent psychiatric disorders.

None of the agents discussed in this chapter are first-line treatments for children, although some have short-term or adjunctive uses. Antidepressants are the long-term treatment of choice for most anxiety disorders in children and adolescents and are discussed in Chapters 4 and 5. Antipsychotics and beta-adrenergic antagonists, which are sometimes used for their sedative and anxiolytic properties, are reviewed in Chapters 7 and 11.

Chemical Properties

Benzodiazepines

Benzodiazepines (BZPs) are unequaled in their ability to acutely reduce anxiety via specific benzodiazepine neuroreceptors (BZP-R). In addition to strong anxiolytic qualities, most benzodiazepines have sedative, muscle-relaxant, and anticonvulsant properties. These properties are linked with the major liability of BZPs: they are potentially addicting. Tolerance develops quickly to their sedative and muscle-relaxant properties. Although tolerance to anxiolytic properties is not as obvious, withdrawal from these drugs does produce anxiety symptoms. This potential problem, and the others discussed below, should make the clinician hesitant to prescribe benzodiazepines for children.

Buspirone

A new category of antianxiety medication, the azapirones, are chemically and clinically distinct from benzodiazepines. Buspirone is currently the only agent available, although several others are under development. Buspirone has no known addictive potential, nor does it cause the cognitive or psychomotor impairment seen with benzodiazepines and antihistamines. Sedative effects are minimal, rendering it ineffective as a hypnotic.

Antihistamines

Although they are widely used for children, there is no specific anxiolytic mechanism postulated for such agents as diphenhydramine (e.g., Benadryl) and hydroxyzine, other than general sedation. However, diphenhydramine is available over the counter and is undoubtably used as a sedative more often than it is prescribed for that purpose. Antihistamines do have other clinically relevant chemical properties, such as the anticholinergic and antiserotonergic activities of diphenhydramine and cyproheptadine respectively. The clinical usefulness of those properties is discussed elsewhere in this handbook.

Indications

Despite FDA approval of benzodiazepines for use in some child and adolescent psychiatric disorders, controlled studies of their efficacy are scarce. Buspirone is still relatively new and unstudied in child and adolescent psychiatry. Antihistamines have long been used as sedatives and hypnotics despite of the absence of convincing data demonstrating their effectiveness.

See Table 10.1.

Anxiety Disorders

Anxiety disorders may have the highest point prevalence of any category of child and adolescent psychiatric illness, 9–17%.[1] Despite this, there are very few controlled pharmacologic trials of childhood anxiety disorders. In fact, nonpharmacologic therapies are the first-line treatment and are effective in the

Table 10.1

**Indications for Sedative and Anxiolytic
Therapy**

Benzodiazepines
Established:
• Panic disorder (short-term)
• Anticipatory anxiety
• Transient primary insomnia (short-term)
• Night terrors
• Acute agitation/violence
Possible:
• Panic disorder (long-term)
• Separation anxiety
• Obsessive-compulsive disorder
• REM behavior disorder
• Mania
Antihistamines
Established:
• Anticipatory anxiety
• Transient primary insomnia
• Acute agitation/violence
Buspirone
Established:
• None
Possible:
• Posttraumatic stress disorder
• Obsessive-compulsive disorder (adjunctive)

majority of cases. When pharmacologic treatment is necessary,
heterocyclic antidepressants and SSRIs are the primary
treatments for panic disorder, separation anxiety, posttraumatic
stress disorder, and obsessive-compulsive disorder (see
Chapters 4 and 5). The anxiolytics discussed in this chapter
either have limited usefulness or have not yet been adequately
tested on children and adolescents.

Panic Disorder
Up to 43% of adolescents report having had at least one panic
attack in their lifetime.[2] Although antidepressants are currently

the pharmacologic treatment of choice (see Chapters 4 and 5), the short-term efficacy of benzodiazepines is well documented in adults. It is likely that benzodiazepines are similarly effective in child and adolescent panic disorder, although their long-term efficacy and adverse effects have not been established. The conservative use of alprazolam as reported by Ballenger and colleagues[3] is a reasonable approach to the general use of benzodiazepines in children. Treatment may be initiated with both alprazolam and a heterocyclic antidepressant so as to provide more rapid relief than would be achieved with an antidepressant alone. Alprazolam may then be tapered after two to three weeks with minimal risk of dependence or withdrawal.[3] Continuing benzodiazepine treatment beyond four weeks may increase the risk of withdrawal anxiety.[4] Alternatively, many clinicians are now choosing an SSRI as first-line pharmacotherapy for panic disorder in children, based more on the superior risk profile of SSRIs than on controlled trials. See Chapter 5 for further discussion of SSRIs. Buspirone has not fared well in controlled trials for adult panic disorder and cannot be recommended for children. Antihistamines have no application in child and adolescent panic disorder.

Separation Anxiety

Separation anxiety accounts for up to half of anxiety-related treatment referrals in children and adolescents.[5] For years, case studies have indicated success in treating separation anxiety with short courses of benzodiazepines. Controlled trials, however, are inconclusive.[1] We recommend exhausting all nonpharmacologic measures before considering any medicine, keeping in mind that the behavioral manifestations of separation anxiety (e.g., school refusal) are usually self-limiting or responsive to psychotherapy. In severe cases where normal function is highly impaired and symptoms persist or escalate, a short course of alprazolam may be useful, but will not replace other treatments. Buspirone essentially has been untested in the treatment of separation anxiety, and antihistamines have no proven role in its treatment.

Generalized Anxiety Disorder

A review of benzodiazepine trials for nonspecific childhood anxiety symptoms suggests that these agents are seldom useful.[6] We recommend considering benzodiazepines in only one such clinical scenario: treatment of anticipatory anxiety prior to a painful procedure. Single doses of short-acting benzodiazepines reduce the psychological trauma of such procedures and are unlikely to produce significant side effects. Buspirone has not been tested sufficiently, outside of periodic case reports, to recommend its use for generalized anxiety disorder in children (formerly, overanxious disorder).

Hydroxyzine, diphenhydramine, and promethazine have been used for nonspecific anxiety symptoms in both children and adults, but have not been well studied. Clinical lore suggests that they are effective in extremely short-term applications, such as for anticipatory anxiety. Since their action is mainly sedative rather than anxiolytic, a single dose of a short-acting benzodiazepine may be more reasonable for this purpose. If an antihistamine is used, we recommend avoiding promethazine, which has produced neuroleptic-like side effects in rare instances (see below).

Posttraumatic Stress Disorder
Most research into posttraumatic stress disorder (PTSD) has been conducted on adult war veterans, but this condition may also affect children exposed to severe trauma, such as sexual abuse, acts of crime and war, or natural disasters. Antidepressants, particularly serotonergic agents, are often helpful, and should be considered first-line therapy (Chapter 5). Benzodiazepines, on the other hand, are usually ineffective and often produce an exacerbation of PTSD symptoms upon withdrawal. We recommend that benzodiazepines be avoided in treating children with PTSD. Neither buspirone nor antihistamines are recommended for this disorder, although buspirone is being tested on adults.

Obsessive-Compulsive Disorder
This potentially devastating anxiety disorder can affect even very young children. The treatment of choice is the SSRIs (see Chapter 5). In general, benzodiazepines are not recommended, although clonazepam may prove an exception to this rule with further testing on children. Buspirone has been used successfully for OCD, as monotherapy and in combination with SSRIs, including in open trials with children and young adults.[7,8] We consider the addition of buspirone a worthwhile

option for youngsters who have shown an incomplete response to SSRIs, although controlled studies are not available and additional improvement in OCD symptoms is often modest.

Insomnia

Insomnia is perhaps the most common problem for which sedatives and anxiolytics are prescribed. Those agents marketed for this purpose are termed hypnotics and are most often antihistamines or short-acting benzodiazepines. Since buspirone produces little or no sedation, it has no application for sleep problems.

Insomnia is most often secondary to a treatable problem, such as a mood disorder, pain, or substance use (caffeine, nicotine, alcohol, etc.). In such cases, the insomnia should be addressed through treatment of the primary disorder. Primary insomnia (that without a definable cause) is an approved indication for hypnotic drugs. However, we do not recommend this use of hypnotics for children and adolescents for several reasons. First, since tolerance develops quickly to the sedative properties of both benzodiazepines and antihistamines, they usually are not effective past one week of therapy. After several weeks of therapy, the risk of rebound insomnia increases and dependence may develop. Second, primary insomnia in childhood is most often related to problems with sleep hygiene, attachment/separation issues, or other psychological factors. Behavioral techniques are usually effective.[9] Finally, in young children, learning to self-initiate and maintain sleep may represent a developmental and behavioral milestone, making nonpharmacologic measures clearly preferable.[10,11]

We recommend that the use of hypnotics in children and adolescents be limited to the rare instances of insomnia caused by psychosocial or physical trauma, travel to a different time zone, or changing from one work shift to another. A reasonable strategy in such instances would be to provide two or three therapeutic doses of a short-acting hypnotic followed by tapering doses over several days. A sedating antihistamine may make more sense in these cases than a benzodiazepine, since the potential for dependence is much lower. A 50-mg dose of diphenhydramine produces sedation roughly equivalent to that provided by 100 mg of pentobarbital.

Parasomnias

Parasomnias are loosely defined as abnormal behaviors during sleep. No studies have tested buspirone for parasomnias, and antihistamines have been reported to exacerbate some cases. However, the relationship of benzodiazepines to three types of parasomnia bears further discussion.

Sleepwalking

Sleepwalking, or somnambulism, appears to be improved in some cases and exacerbated in others by treatment with benzodiazepines. We do not recommend treatment with benzodiazepines, since the clinical course is usually benign and safety can nearly always be ensured with environmental controls.

Night Terrors

Night terrors, or pavor nocturnus, consist of the sudden onset of intense fear and autonomic discharge, usually occurring during slow-wave sleep. The child screams, is confused and inconsolable, and may cause injury by bolting from his or her bed. Environmental measures, supportive psychotherapy, and improved sleep habits are usually sufficient, but short-term hypnotic therapy may be used in severe cases. Midazolam, 15 mg at the hour of sleep, appears to be particularly effective, although its long-term efficacy is untested. To minimize tolerance, hypnotic therapy of night terrors should be limited to short-term, intermittent courses.

REM Behavior Disorder

Rapid-eye-movement (REM) behavior disorder is a rare and unusual syndrome that generally appears in adults, but has also been reported in children.[12] The syndrome is characterized by the maintenance of muscle tone during REM sleep, causing elaborate, seemingly purposeful, behavior. Most pharmacologic data come from a single research center, where the syndrome has been successfully managed with clonazepam. There is no consensus regarding treatment of this rare syndrome in children.

Aggression

Benzodiazepines and antihistamines are frequently used to manage acute episodes of violence or agitation in pediatric inpatient settings. Although this is a logical application for sedative agents, it is not an approved indication for benzodiazepines or antihistamines. Still, such agents as lorazepam, midazolam, and diphenhydramine given IM are effective in many cases. Clearly, they are safer than sedating antipsychotics, which are approved for this use (see Chapter 7).

In general, the authors prefer first-line use of IM lorazepam or diphenhydramine for mild to moderate agitation when pharmacologic treatment is unavoidable. However, the clinician must also be aware that a significant number of children will have a disinhibitory response to benzodiazepines (see Table 10.3). Interestingly, Vitiello and associates[13] found that administering an IM agent to agitated children had a calming effect, whether that agent was diphenhydramine or placebo.

Neither benzodiazepines nor antihistamines are recommended for the management of chronic aggression. However, buspirone has been reported to improve such states. It may be reasonable to try buspirone in aggressive children when lithium and beta-adrenergic agents have failed. The risks of buspirone treatment are far preferable to those of anticonvulsants or antipsychotics.

Bipolar Affective Disorder

Clonazepam and lorazepam have emerged as probable antimanic agents in the treatment of adult bipolar affective disorder, used both in combination with lithium and as single agents. No comparable studies have been performed on children, but clonazepam may be tried in refractory cases.

Contraindications

See Table 10.2.

Benzodiazepines

Agents that undergo hepatic metabolism are to be avoided in patients with hepatic dysfunction. Temazepam and oxazepam, for example, do not undergo hepatic metabolism. Patients treated with any benzodiazepine must be cautioned against driving or performing dangerous tasks, especially early in therapy.

Buspirone

Because buspirone has significant serotonergic activity, it may induce a central excitatory syndrome, or "serotonin syndrome," if used concurrently with MAOIs.

Table 10.2

Contraindications to Sedative and Anxiolytic Therapy

Benzodiazepines
Absolute:
• Prior hypersensitivity reaction
• Narrow-angle glaucoma (most agents)
Relative:
• Prior disinhibitory reactions
• Dependence on or abuse of benzodiazepines and related substances
• Hepatic dysfunction (some agents)
• Patients at risk for falls or aspiration
• Patients with AIDS receiving zidovudine
• Patients with symptomatic sleep apnea
Antihistamines
Absolute:
• Prior hypersensitivity reaction
• Narrow-angle glaucoma (anticholinergic agents)
Relative:
• Gastrointestinal or urinary obstructions (anticholinergic agents)
• Signs or risk of anticholinergic toxicity (anticholinergic agents)
• Patients taking other CNS depressants or analgesics
Buspirone
Absolute:
• Prior hypersensitivity reaction
• Concurrent treatment with MAOIs
Relative:
• Patients with hepatic or renal dysfunction

Antihistamines

Diphenhydramine and cyproheptadine are particularly anticholinergic and should be avoided when these effects would be undesirable. In addition, most antihistamines potentiate other CNS depressants and analgesics, necessitating caution when combined with these agents. Like benzodiazepines, such agents may cause impairment of driving or work performance and patients must be so cautioned.

Side Effects

See Table 10.3.

Table 10.3

Side Effects of Sedative and Anxiolytic Therapy

Benzodiazepines
Common:
   • Sedation
   • Decreased cognitive and psychomotor performance
   • Disinhibitory reactions
Rare:
   • Seizures (with abrupt withdrawal)

Antihistamines
Common:
   • Sedation
   • Dizziness
   • Gastrointestinal upset
   • Anticholinergic side effects (diphenhydramine and cyproheptadine)
Rare:
   • Lowered seizure threshold
   • Hypotension
   • Tachycardia
   • Blood dyscrasias
   • Involuntary movement disorders (at high doses)

Buspirone
Common:
   • Dizziness
   • Insomnia
   • Sedation or fatigue (mild)
   • Gastrointestinal upset
   • Headache
   • Irritability or excitement
Rare:
   • No serious adverse effects reported

Benzodiazepines

Although tolerance to sedation develops rapidly, the effects of benzodiazepines on cognitive and psychomotor performance may persist at low levels.[14,15] This is of obvious concern in school-age children and represents a major risk of benzodiazepine therapy in this age group. A lesser risk, but one that must be considered, is that of disinhibitory reactions. Its frequency in developmentally normal children is unknown, but may be as high as 10% in children with some degree of neurologic impairment. With high doses, such as those used for presurgical sedation and acute agitation, the incidence may be as high as 23%, even among healthy children and adolescents.[16,17] A final, potentially serious effect of benzodiazepine treatment is withdrawal seizures. The risk is greatest when high doses of short-acting agents are stopped abruptly, but the precise incidence is unknown.

Antihistamines and Buspirone

These medications generally have few serious side effects, although minor side effects can be quite unpleasant (Table 10.3). Anticholinergic effects of antihistamines include dry mouth, constipation, urinary retention, blurred vision, and confusion. Promethazine has weak antidopamine activity and at high doses can produce a full range of antipsychotic side effects, including dystonia and involuntary movement disorders.

Overdose

Benzodiazepines

The symptoms of benzodiazepine toxicity include drowsiness, ataxia, confusion, slurred speech, tremor, and diplopia. Respiratory depression can occur, but is rare. In extreme cases, bradycardia and coma may result. Visual and tactile hallucinations have been reported in children experiencing benzodiazepine toxicity.[18]

Buspirone

Buspirone toxicity consists of more severe forms of gastric distress and miosis. No deaths have been reported as a result of buspirone overdose.

Antihistamine

Antihistamine overdose is associated with sedation, hypotension, and, for some agents, anticholinergic toxicity and delirium. The anticholinesterase physostigmine may be used as an antidote to anticholinergic toxicity in severe cases.

Abuse/Dependence

Benzodiazepines

Benzodiazepines are among the most frequently abused prescription medications,[19] with the greatest risk found among alcoholic patients.[20] The short-acting agents are the most likely to be abused. Illicitly acquired benzodiazepines are used recreationally by adolescents, but the prevalence of the practice in the United States has not been studied. In contrast, antihistamines and buspirone are not commonly abused, although tolerance does develop to antihistamines. No withdrawal syndrome has been described for antihistamines or buspirone.

Drug Interactions

See Table 10.4.

Clinical Practice

Benzodiazepines

Since benzodiazepines have limited utility in child and adolescent psychiatric disorders, precise clinical guidelines for their use have not been established. However, basic guidelines are offered in Table 10.5, based on recommendations by Coffey,[21] the experience of the authors, and additional published reports.

No specific premedication laboratory evaluation is needed to initiate benzodiazepine treatment. For dosing in young children, it may be necessary to cut tablets into quarters for some medications. For sleep induction, a reasonable dose for short-acting hypnotics is one half of the adult starting dose for preadolescent children and the lower limit of the adult dose for adolescents. Unless the clinician is considering long-term (unproven) treatment of bipolar disorder or OCD, benzodiazepine therapy for children and adolescents should be of short duration: less than 30 days for panic disorder and less than two weeks for insomnia. This approach minimizes the risk of dependence, as well as any cognitive and psychomotor side effects.

Several strategies for withdrawal of benzodiazepine treatment have been advocated. Single-dose or intermittent single-dose prescription may require no special withdrawal program, but patients should be warned about rebound insomnia even in these cases. If the benzodiazepine has been taken chronically, then a gradual taper is recommended and may take weeks or months. Since the risk of severe withdrawal is greatest with short-acting compounds, it may be useful to switch to a

Table 10.4

Drug Interactions with Anxiolytics and Sedatives

Benzodiazepines

Drugs potentiated by benzodiazepines:
- Alcohol
- Sedatives (narcotic, analgesic, recreational)
- Tricyclic antidepressants
- Phenytoin
- Zidovudine

Drugs that potentiate benzodiazepines:
- Antimicrobials (erythromycin, isoniazid)
- Oral contraceptives
- Cimetidine
- Alcohol
- Sedatives
- Neuroleptics
- MAOIs

Drugs whose activity may be impaired:
- Carbamazepine

Drugs that inhibit activity of benzodiazepines:
- Antacids

Drugs that may produce adverse reactions:
- MAOIs (central excitatory syndrome)

Antihistamines

Drugs potentiated by antihistamines:
- Alcohol
- Sedatives (narcotic, analgesic, recreational)

Drugs that may produce adverse reactions:
- Potentiation of anticholinergic side effects and possible toxicity with any anticholinergic agent

Buspirone

Drugs potentiated by buspirone:
- Neuroleptics (theoretical and one report of increased haloperidol levels)

Drugs that may produce adverse reactions:
- Trazodone (one report of hepatic toxicity)
- MAOIs (theoretical risk of central excitatory syndrome)
- Neuroleptics (theoretical risk of increased effects of dopamine antagonism)

Table 10.5

Suggested Agents and Dosing Guidelines for the Use of Sedative/Anxiolytic Agents for Children and Adolescents

Indication	Suggested Agents	Starting Doses		Maximum Daily Dose	
		Preadolescent	Adolescent	Preadolescent	Adolescent
Panic disorder	Alprazolam	0.125 mg b.i.d. or t.i.d	0.25 mg b.i.d. or t.i.d	1–4 mg	8–10 mg
	Clonazepam	0.25 mg q.d.	0.5 mg q.d.	0.1–0.2 mg/kg*	0.1–0.2 mg/kg*
Anticipatory anxiety	Alprazolam	0.125–0.25 mg	0.25–0.5 mg	NA	NA
	Diphenhydramine	25–50 mg	50–100 mg	5 mg/kg	5 mg/kg
	Hydroxyzine	0.6 mg/kg	0.6 mg/kg	NA	NA
Overanxious disorder	Buspirone	2.5 mg b.i.d.	5 mg b.i.d.	20 mg/day	60 mg/day
Insomnia	Diphenhydramine	25–50 mg 50% of adult starting dose	50–100 mg Lower limit of adult dose	5 mg/kg 50% of adult maximum	5 mg/kg Adult maximum
	Any short-acting benzodiazepine hypnotic				

*Dose is the maximum recommended for seizure disorders; not established for psychiatric indications.

long-acting agent, such as diazepam or clonazepam at equivalent potency, before tapering the drug.

See Table 10.5

Buspirone

Buspirone is likewise without guidelines for children and has not been approved for use for those under the age of 18. Again, no specific laboratory tests are necessary. If used for anxiety disorders, we suggest titrating (increments as small as 2.5 mg) to a divided daily dose of 5 to 15 mg for preadolescents and 20 mg for adolescents. Thereafter, dosing should be based on clinical response and side effects. The optimal dose for the treatment of chronic aggression may be 50% lower than for anxiety disorders. Minor side effects of buspirone may be addressed symptomatically or by lowering the dose.

Antihistamines

There is little or no evidence supporting the use of antihistamines in the treatment of anxiety disorders. The two most appropriate indications are insomnia and situational or anticipatory anxiety. These situations require single doses or very brief courses of treatment, the dosing guidelines for which appear in Table 10.5. Since these medications are recommended only for short-term use, side effects are generally tolerable.

References

1. Bernstein, G.A., Borchardt, C.M. (1991). Anxiety disorders of childhood and adolescence: A critical review. *J Am Acad Child Adolesc Psychiatry*, *30*, 519–532.
2. King, N.J., Gullone, E., Tonge, B.J., Ollendick, T.H. (1993). Self-reports of panic attacks and manifest anxiety in adolescents. *Behav Res Ther*, *31*, 111–116.
3. Ballenger, J.C., Carek, D.J., Steele, J.J., Cornish-McTighe, D. (1989). Three cases of panic disorder with agoraphobia in children. *Am J Psychiatry*, *146*, 922–924.
4. Woods, S.W., Nagy, L.M., Koleszar, A.S., et al.(1992). Controlled trial of alprazolam supplementation during imipramine treatment of panic disorder. *J Clin Psychopharmacology*, *12*, 32–38.
5. Last, C.G., Perrin, S., Hersen, M., Kazdin, A.E. (1992). DSM-III-R anxiety disorders in children: Sociodemographic and clinical characteristics. *J Am Acad Child Adolesc Psychiatry*, *31*, 1070–1076.

6. Rosenberg, D.R., Holttum, J., Gershon, S. (Eds.) (1994). *Textbook of Pharmacotherapy for Child and Adolescent Psychiatric Disorders*. New York: Brunner/Mazel.

7. Alessi, N., Bos, T. (1991). Buspirone augmentation of fluoxetine in a depressed child with obsessive-compulsive disorder. *Am J Psychiatry, 148*, 1605–1606.

8. Markovitz, P.J., Stagno, S.J., Calabrese, J.R. (1990). Buspirone augmentation of fluoxetine in obsessive-compulsive disorder. *Am J Psychiatry, 147*, 798–800.

9. Bootzin, R.R., Perlis, M.L. (1992). Nonpharmacologic treatments of insomnia. *J Clin Psychiatry, 53(6 suppl.)*, 37–41.

10. Dahl, R.E. (1992). The pharmacologic treatment of sleep disorders. *Pediatr Psychopharmacol, 15*, 161–178.

11. Durand, V.M., Mindell, J.A. (1990). Behavioral treatment of multiple childhood sleep disorders. Effects on child and family. *Behav Modif, 14*, 37–49.

12. Schenck, C.H., et al. (1986). REM behavior disorder in a 10-year old girl and aperiodic TEM and NREM sleep movements in an 8-year old brother. *Sleep Res, 15*, 162.

13. Vitiello, B., Hill, J.L., Elia, J., et al. (1991). P.r.n. medications in child psychiatric patients: A pilot placebo-controlled study. *J Clin Psychiatry, 52*, 499–501.

14. Johnson, L.C., Chernik, D.A. (1982). Sedative-hypnotics and human performance. *Psychopharmacology, 76*, 101–113.

15. Sakol, M.S., Power, K.G. (1988). The effects of long-term benzodiazepine treatment and graded withdrawal on psychometric performance. *Psychopharmacology, 95*, 135–138.

16. Litchfield, B.N. (1980). Complications of intravenous dizepam—adverse psychological reactions (an assessment of 16,000 cases). *Anesth Prog, 27*, 175.

17. Roelofse, J.A., van der Bijl, P., Stegmann, D.H., et al. (1990). Preanesthetic medication with rectal midazolam in children undergoing dental extractions. *J Oral Maxillofac Surg, 48*, 791.

18. Pfefferbaum, B., Butler, P.M., Mullins, D., Copeland, D.R. (1987). Two cases of benzodiazepine toxicity in children. *J Clin Psychiatry, 48*, 450–452.

19. Wolf, B., Grohmann, R., Biber, D., et al. (1989). Benzodiazepine abuse and dependence in psychiatric inpatients. *Pharmacopsychiatry, 22*, 54–60.

20. Ciraulo, D.A., Sands, B.F., Shader, R.I. (1988). Critical review of liability for benzodiazepine abuse among alcoholics. *Am J Psychiatry, 145*, 1501–1506.

21. Coffey, B. (1990). Anxiolytics for children and adolescents: Traditional and new drugs. *J Child Adolesc Psychopharmacol, 1*, 57–83.

C h a p t e r 11

Adrenergic Agents in Child and Adolescent Psychiatry

Clonidine

Clonidine is an alpha-2-adrenergic agonist with antihypertensive efficacy and is currently under investigation to better delineate its role in the pharmacotherapy of children and adolescents with psychiatric disorders. It has been most studied in pediatric patients with Tourette's syndrome and ADHD. Clonidine is most effective in decreasing hyperarousal and motoric overactivity, and less efficacious in reducing distractibility and improving decreased attention span.[1]

Chemical Properties

See Table 11.1.

Through its alpha-2-adrenergic receptor agonist activity, clonidine affects the locus ceruleus, the major noradrenergic center in the brain, resulting in a decrease in the amount of this type of neurotransmitter being released from the nerve terminal. Oral clonidine is almost completely absorbed from the GI tract, with a rapid onset of action. Clonidine's behavioral effects last between three and six hours, while sedative effects are most prominent 30 to 90 minutes after the last dose, in contrast to its antihypertensive and cardiac effects, which begin within 30 to 60 minutes of ingestion and last for six to eight hours. Clonidine is also available as a skin patch known as the transdermal system. In children, the behavioral effects are often noted within two to three days of applying the skin patch;

Table 11.1

Pharmacokinetics of Adrenergic Agents in Children and Adolescents

Generic Name (Brand Name)	Selectivity	Peak Plasma Concentration (hours)	Plasma Half-Life (hours)	Metabolism and Excretion	Comments
Clonidine (Catapres)	Alpha-2	1–3	8–12	35% hepatic and 65% renal	Very lipophilic; easily penetrates blood-brain barrier
Propranolol (Inderal)	None	1–1½	4	Hepatic	Very lipophilic; potent central and peripheral effects
Atenolol (Tenormin)	Beta-1 (higher doses affects β-2 also)	2–4	6–7	Renal	May be better tolerated than propranolol by children with fewer side effects
Guanfacine (Tenex)	Alpha-2	1–4	17 (10–30)	Renal	May be better tolerated by children and adolescents than clonidine with fewer side effects

Table 11.2

Indications for Clonidine in Psychiatry

FDA-Approved Indications: • None
Likely Indications: • Tourette's disorder • ADHD in children and adolescents • Opioid withdrawal • Nicotine withdrawal
Possible Indications: • Anxiety and panic disorders • Bipolar disorder in children and adolescents • Psychosis • Agitation (anxiety, hyperarousal) • Neuroleptic-induced akathisia • ADHD in adults • Borderline personality disorder • Social phobia • PTSD

this corresponds to its maximal antihypertensive effect, which occurs two to three days after it is initiated.

Indications

See Table 11.2.

Tourette's Syndrome

Although clonidine appears to be less effective than neuroleptics in the treatment of Tourette's syndrome, it still is a useful treatment, with many patients showing a 50% or greater decrease in their symptoms.[2-5] A major advantage of clonidine is that it does not incur the long-term side effects associated with neuroleptic use, such as tardive dyskinesia. Clonidine has also been found to be effective in decreasing the symptoms of tic disorder during haloperidol withdrawal. It enhances the efficacy of neuroleptics in the treatment of Tourette's syndrome, allowing for the use of lower doses of neuroleptics. It should be noted that haloperidol has been shown to be more effective than clonazepam, which is in turn more effective than clonidine in treating patients with Tourette's syndrome. Because of the severe adverse side effects associated with neuroleptic use, we recommend using clonazepam as the initial treatment for Tourette's syndrome, followed by a combination of clonazepam and clonidine. Clonidine appears to be especially helpful in certain subgroups of patients, including those with mild tics and obsessive-compulsive symptoms and with comorbid ADHD and Tourette's syndrome.[6-9] Clonidine and methylphenidate have also been used to treat comorbid ADHD and Tourette's syndrome, although many clinicians consider Tourette's syndrome an absolute contraindication to stimulant use (see Chapter 3, Psychostimulants).

Attention-Deficit/Hyperactivity Disorder
Clonidine has been shown to be effective in the treatment of disruptive behavior in children and adolescents. The most clonidine-sensitive children appear to be those with high rates of motoric hyperactivity, coexistent oppositional or conduct disorders, and onset of their symptoms at an early age. Clonidine decreases motor overactivity and hyperarousal states and improves frustration tolerance in these children, often leading to their increased compliance with commands and expectations of better learning and improved grades. It is not effective in patients with ADHD when the primary problem is distractibility and decreased attention span. Methylphenidate is more effective than clonidine in improving distractibility and attention difficulties.

Opioid Withdrawal
Clonidine has been successful in helping adults withdraw from narcotics,[10] but has not been well studied in children and adolescents. Children and adolescents require pharmacologic treatment for drug and alcohol withdrawal far less commonly than do adults. Moreover, withdrawal from narcotics, although uncomfortable, is not lethal as is the case with barbiturates. If its use is deemed necessary due to unusual circumstances, we advise consultation with an expert in the field of addiction, and the application of, adult guidelines, with modifications for younger populations as indicated. In adults, doses of 0.15 mg b.i.d. are used for opioid withdrawal.

Posttraumatic Stress Disorder

In adults with PTSD, clonidine has been shown to reduce anxiety, hyperarousal, and intense and intrusive flashbacks of the precipitating trauma, but not avoidant-type behaviors. As there are no data on children and adolescents, we do not recommend the use of clonidine for PTSD in pediatric patients.

Social Phobia

Clonidine has been moderately effective in treating some adults with social phobia. As there are no data on this medication in children, we do not recommend its use in treating social phobia in children and adolescents.

Contraindications

See Table 11.3.

There are no absolute contraindications to clonidine's use. However, it should generally be avoided for children and adolescents with depression, cardiovascular disorders, renal disease, a history of allergic reactions to clonidine, skin irritation or disease (skin patch only), liver disease, and those who are pregnant.

Side Effects

See Table 11.4.

Sedation, the most common side effect that children and adolescents experience while on clonidine, is most noticeable and problematic during the first month of treatment, but

Table 11.3

Contraindications to Clonidine Use

Absolute:
• None
Relative:
• Depression (in patient or family history)
• Cardiovascular disorders
• Renal or liver disease
• Skin disease/irritation (for skin patch only)
• Pregnancy

Table 11.4

Side Effects of Clonidine

Common:
- Sedation
- Hypotension
- Cardiovascular
- Headache and dizziness
- Stomachache/nausea/vomiting

Uncommon:
- Depression
- Cardiac arrhythmias
- Rebound hypertension
- Retinal degeneration
- Skin irritation with skin patch
- Anticholinergic
- Vivid dreams/nightmares/disrupted sleep
- Appetite increase or decrease
- Sexual dysfunction
- Fluid retention
- Anxiety
- Increased blood glucose
- Raynaud's phenomenon

usually remits progressively thereafter. In 15% of children on clonidine, however, the sedation persists, and in 10%, even dose adjustment is not successful in decreasing it and the medication must be discontinued. Hypotension is a common side effect of clonidine therapy in children and adolescents, with children often experiencing a 10% reduction in systolic blood pressure. This is rarely clinically significant. Sedation correlates with decreased blood pressure.

Cardiovascular side effects are not uncommon in pediatric patients treated with clonidine, but these rarely are clinically significant. Clonidine acutely decreases cardiac output by 10 to 20%, but chronically, cardiac output returns to baseline. Clonidine causes depression in 5% of children and adolescents treated with this medication, but most of these have significant depressive symptoms at the start of clonidine treatment, as well as a personal or family history of mood disorders. Headache, dizziness, stomachache, nausea, and vomiting are common side effects observed during the first month of clonidine treatment, and are most often short-term effects that dissipate after the first month. Uncommon side effects of clonidine include cardiac arrhythmias, rebound hypertension, retinal degeneration, skin irritation with skin patch, anticholinergic effects, nightmares, appetite change, sexual dysfunction, fluid retention, anxiety, increased blood glucose, and Raynaud's phenomenon.

Drug Interactions

See Table 11.5.

Clinical Practice

For the dosing and administration of clonidine, see Table 11.6.

See Table 11.6.

Prior to initiating clonidine therapy, children and adolescents must have a comprehensive baseline history and a physical examination documenting blood pressure and pulse measurements. Careful screening for depression in the patient and family is indicated as its presence contraindicates clonidine's use. The clinician should also obtain baseline CBC and differential, electrolytes, BUN and creatinine, thyroid function tests, liver function tests, ECG, and fasting blood glucose. While the patient is on clonidine, orthostatic measurements of blood pressure and pulse should be obtained weekly until the dose is stabilized, after which they should be monitored every two months. More frequent monitoring is indicated if the patient experiences sedation, as blood pressure and sedation have been found to correlate with each other.

When the decision is made to discontinue clonidine, it is essential that it be withdrawn gradually. In children, if clonidine has been prescribed for less than one week, abrupt discontinuation of the 0.05-mg bedtime dose does not usually result in rebound hypertension or other problems. When clonidine has been given for two to three weeks, gradual tapering by 0.05 mg/day is recommended. After the child has been on clonidine for one month or longer, clonidine should be reduced by 0.05 mg every three to seven days. Finally, if a child or adolescent is on both clonidine and a beta-blocker, such as

Table 11.5

Clonidine and Guanfacine Interactions

*Increases Drug Effect of:

- Heterocyclic antidepressants
- Antipsychotics
- Anticholinergic medications
- CNS depressants (i.e., alcohol)

*Decreases Drug Effect of:

- Beta-blockers

*Increases Effect of Clonidine:

- Fenfluramine
- Diuretics
- Other antihypertensive medications
- CNS depressants

*Decreases Effect of Clonidine:

- Heterocyclic antidepressants
- Sympathomimetic drugs
- Nonsteroidal anti-inflammatory analgesics

*Increases Levels of:

- Growth hormone levels (short-term)
- Blood glucose

*Decreases Levels of:

- Urinary catecholamines

*May Cause:

- Abnormal liver function tests
- Wenckebach periods on ventricular trigeminy

* May be less with guanfacine.
Adapted from: Lowenthai, D.T. Matzek, K.M., MacGregor, T.R. (1988). Clinical pharmacokinetics of clonidine. *Clin Pharmacokinet, 14,* 287–310.

Table 11.6

Clinician's Guide to Using Clonidine for Tourette's Disorder and ADHD in Children and Adolescents

Tourette's Disorder	ADHD
• Start with 0.05 mg at bedtime, increase by 0.05 mg every three to seven days • Optimal dose 3–4 μg/kg/day, three to four times a day (after meals and at bedtime) • After stable oral dose achieved, may switch to skin patch (same dose) • Not FDA-approved	• Start with 0.05 mg at bedtime, increase by 0.05 mg every three to seven days • Optimal dose 3–6 μg/kg/day • After stable oral dose, may switch to skin patch • Not FDA-approved

propranolol, the beta-blocker should be discontinued several days before initiating the clonidine taper in order to avoid rebound hypertension.

In addition to an oral form, clonidine is also available as a skin patch (transdermal system). In children, the behavioral effects are noted within two to three days of applying the patch. The clonidine skin patch is available as Catapres-TTS 1, 2, and 3, which correspond to oral clonidine doses of 0.1, 0.2, and 0.3 mg. Cutting the patch can produce intermediate doses so that oral doses can be duplicated with the skin patch. It is not advisable to start clonidine treatment with the skin patch because oral clonidine can be used more easily to determine treatment response, making the switch to an equivalent dose of transdermal clonidine easier. Absorption via the skin patch is more variable than after the oral administration of clonidine. There is no fixed ratio of doses between routes of administration.

When selecting the site for application of the clonidine patch on children and adolescents, choose an inaccessible area without hair on the lower back. Prepare the skin by washing with soap and water and then drying. Apply the patch to the designated area, much like a Band Aid. Place a 3-cm white adhesive strip over the patch to make sure that it stays on. The clonidine skin

Table 11.7

Clonidine Overdose

Signs and Symptoms:
- Decreased or absent reflexes
- Lethargy or somnolence
- Dilated pupils
- Hypotension
- Irritability
- Seizures
- Apnea
- Reversible cardiac conduction defects and arrhythmias

Treatment of Overdose:
- Remove all clonidine systems, such as skin patch
- IV fluids and/or pressors to treat hypotension
- Atropine for bradycardia
- Careful monitoring of the patient's respiratory status

---

patch is resilient to brief water exposure and does not have to be replaced after a shower or bath, but it may require replacement on very humid days or when the child has been swimming for an entire day. The patch is effective for five days and should be replaced after this time. Nonspecific sedation is often noticed soon after the patch is initiated. Clinical response is rarely observed before two weeks of treatment.

Overdose

Clonidine overdose can be a life-threatening clinical emergency that can result in death. See Table 11.7.

Abuse

Clonidine has a very low risk for abuse.

Guanfacine Hydrochloride

Recently, another centrally acting antihypertensive alpha-2 adrenoreceptor agonist, guanfacine hydrochloride (Tenex) has been utilized to treat the same neuropsychiatric disorders for which clonidine has been use (see above). Its plasma half-life is approximately 17 hours. Peak plasma levels occur within two to three hours of administration and steady state blood levels are typically achieved within four to five days. Its side-effect profile is similar to clonidine, although preliminary study suggests that guanfacine may be less sedating than clonidine and be more easily tolerated in general by pediatric patients. In addition, unlike clonidine, there have been no reported cases of cardiac toxicity or death with guanfacine-methylphenidate combinations, although this medication has not been used as commonly as clonidine. While not FDA-approved for any psychiatric conditions, below we list its major possible indications and dosing strategies.

Attention-Deficit/Hyperactivity Disorder/Tourette's Syndrome
There have been no controlled studies of guanfacine in ADHA or Tourette's Syndrome. Open studies suggest that it can be effective in both conditions.[11,12,13] It also appears to be better tolerated than clonidine by many children with fewer side effects, particularly sedation. Moreover, guanfacine may also be effective in ameliorating inattentiveness and distractibility, while clonidine typically is effective in reducing motoric hyperactivity but ineffective in improving attention and reducing distractibility. Mean optimal doses of 3.5 mg per day appear to be most effective in ameliorating target symptoms. The recommended dosing strategy is to start guanfacine at 0.5 mg (1/2 pill) per day and then increase the dose by 0.5 mg (1/2 pill) every three days to a maximum of 4 mg per day. A dose of 3.5 mg per day appears to be the most capable of achieving maximal efficacy with minimal toxicity. This dosage is given in divided doses of 0.5 mg at breakfast, 0.5 mg at lunch, 0.5 mg at 4 p.m. and 1 mg at bedtime.

Propranolol

Beta-Blockers

The beta-blockers competitively antagonize epinephrine and norepinephrine activity at the beta-adrenergic receptors. They have no FDA-established indications for use in psychiatric disorders. Propranolol is a nonselective beta-1 and beta-2 antagonist, and has been the most investigated agent of its class, so we will focus on this agent in this chapter. There is evidence that propranolol is effective in the treatment of aggressive patients with organic brain disease. It has also been reported to

Table 11.8

Pharmacokinetic Properties of Propranolol (in Adults)

Drug (Brand Name)	Selectivity	Lipophilicity	Peak Effect (Hours)	Plasma Half-Life (Hours)	Elimi- nation
Propranolol (Inderal)	None	High	1–1 $\frac{1}{2}$	3–6	Hepatic

be effective in treating panic disorder, PTSD, performance anxiety, social phobia, and akathisia. Its ability to decrease anxiety and agitation in specific psychiatric disorders appears to be due to its peripheral actions of slowing the increased heart rate associated with anxiety and hyperarousal rather than to its central effects on beta adrenergic receptors. Some clinicians use propranolol to treat children and adolescents with impulsivity and aggression, particularly when there is CNS damage, such as mental retardation, or when such patients have failed first-line treatments of disruptive behavior disorders.

Chemical Properties

See Table 11.8.

The mechanism by which propranolol is effective in the treatment of anxiety and hyperarousal states has not been clearly established. Propranolol blocks both beta-1 and beta-2 receptors in the brain and peripheral nervous system. It blocks the actions of norepinephrine and epinephrine at these receptors. Since norepinephrine and epinephrine are associated with sympathetic arousal, propranolol exerts sympatholytic effects, such as reducing heart rate and blood pressure.

Indications

See Table 11.9.

Aggressive Children and Adolescents with CNS Disease
Propranolol has been reported to be effective in the treatment of violent behavior in adult patients with organic brain disease. Subsequently, open-label studies have suggested that children and adolescents with uncontrollable rage and aggressive outbursts experience moderate to marked improvement when

Table 11.9

Indications for Propranolol for Children and Adolescents

FDA-Established Indications: • None
Possible Indications: • Aggressive patients with CNS damage • Akathisia • Alcohol withdrawal • Generalized anxiety disorder and panic disorder • Hyperventilation attacks • Lithium tremor • Performance anxiety • PTSD
Not Indicated: • Extrapyramidal side effects of neuroleptics (except akathisia) • Schizophrenia • Tardive dyskinesia

treated with propranolol. Median doses of 160 mg of propranolol per day are required. Side effects have been reported to be minimal, even at higher doses, in children treated with propranolol.

Akathisia

Many clinicians believe that beta-blockers, such as propranolol, are the drugs of choice for neuroleptic-induced akathisia in adults. In children, where it is often difficult to differentiate akathisia from hyperactivity. Conservative measures such as adjusting the antipsychotic medication dosage, are preferred.

Performance Anxiety

Propranolol has been reported to be effective in improving performance anxiety in adults; for example, a single dose of 10 to 40 mg of propranolol 30 to 60 minutes before the anxiety-producing event. It is wise to give the patient a test dose prior to a very important event to make sure that it will help and that it will not cause problematic side effects. Adolescents have been reported to have improved scores on

Scholastic Aptitude Tests after taking propranolol. The authors have found that low doses of propranolol (e.g., a single 10-mg dose) taken 30 to 60 minutes before a school examination can improve the performance of children and adolescents with severe test-taking anxiety that has been refractory to all behavioral and nonchemical interventions, but is not due to cognitive impairment. Starting with a dose of 10 mg is recommended. If the child shows the desired improved performance, using this medication prior to subsequent tests or having it available as needed for the child is recommended. Side effects, such as dizziness, hypotension, or forgetfulness, require its discontinuation or a reduction to the previously tolerated dose. We also recommend testing each dose increase prior to the important event or examination.

Posttraumatic Stress Disorder
Propranolol initiated in open-label fashion at 0.8 mg/kg/day and increased gradually to a maximum of 2.5 mg/kg/day has been shown to be effective in treating hyperaroused, treatment-refractory PTSD children. Maintaining dosages at this level for two weeks, and then gradually discontinuing the medication over the next three weeks has been reported to result in continued good functioning without the relapse of symptoms. It is possible that doses of beta-blockers lower than those used in the treatment of anxiety disorders may be effective in treating acute PTSD, and that as-needed doses prior to stressful situations may be especially helpful. Further study is required, but this appears to be a promising intervention for children and adolescents suffering from PTSD.

Contraindications
See Table 11.10.

Absolute contraindications to propranolol's use include patients with bronchospastic disease (such as asthma), or cardiovascular disease, as well as those on MAOIs having a known hypersensitivity or history of allergic reaction to beta-blockers. Propranolol should also be avoided in patients with uncontrolled diabetes, with hyperthyroidism or depression or who are pregnant.

Side Effects
See Table 11.11.

Table 11.10

Contraindications to Propranolol Use

- Bronchospastic disease (asthma)
- Diabetes/hypoglycemia
- Allergic reaction
- Medicated with MAOI
- Hyperthyroidism
- Depression
- Pregnancy

Table 11.11

Side Effects of Propranolol

Common:
- Decreased heart rate
- Raynaud's phenomenon
- Lethargy
- Impotence

Uncommon:
- Bronchoconstriction
- Congestive heart failure
- Depression
- Hallucinations

Rare:
- Hypoglycemia
- Hypotension/dizziness
- Nausea/diarrhea
- Vivid dreams and nightmares

It is critical to get baseline vital signs and to monitor cardiac function while children and adolescents are receiving propranolol, as this medication can decrease the pulse rate to less than 50 beats per minute. Starting at low doses of propranolol, such as 10 mg/day, and increasing them gradually are recommended. Decreased pulse rate is much less common when atenolol is used instead of propranolol. Raynaud's phenomenon, tiredness and weakness, and sexual impotence are common side effects of propranolol. Bronchoconstriction is an uncommon but potentially life-threatening side effect of propranolol that is even less common with atenolol. However, we recommend immediate discontinuation of all beta-blockers when this side effect is observed. Depression is another uncommon but potentially severe side effect of propranolol treatment, that also appears to be less common when atenolol is used instead. We recommend discontinuing propranolol on depressed patients and switching to atenolol. We specifically do not agree with the view of some clinicians that depression induced by propranolol can be treated with an antidepressant instead of discontinuing the propranolol. Beta-blockers mask symptoms of hypoglycemia, complicating treatment of diabetes. Hallucinations are an uncommon side effect of propranolol that are believed to be nonexistent in patients treated with atenolol. Rare side effects of propranolol include hypoglycemia, hypotension, dizziness, nausea and diarrhea, and nightmares. Nightmares and sleep disturbances appear to be almost nonexistent with beta-blockers other than propranolol, such as atenolol.

Drug Interactions

See Table 11.12.

Clinical Practice

See Table 11.13.

Prior to initiating propranolol, children and adolescents should have a physical examination with measurement of heart rate and blood pressure. An ECG should be performed. Screening for bronchospastic illness, such as asthma, is required. If such an illness is present, propranolol use is contraindicated. A pregnancy test and evaluation for adequate contraceptive use is advised for females of childbearing age. Males and females should be informed of the risk for sexual dysfunction with propranolol, since this is a relatively common side effect. Start with low-dose propranolol, 10 mg/day, and increase the dose gradually to ensure that the blood pressure and pulse rate drop as little as possible. If the blood pressure decreases to below 90/60 mmHg and/or if the pulse rate falls to less than 60 beats

Table 11.12

Drug Interactions

Propranolol may Increase Effects of:
• Anesthetics
• Antipsychotics
• Calcium blockers
• Clonidine
• Epinephrine
• Lidocaine
• MAOIs
• Phenytoin
• Thyroxine
Propranolol may Decrease Effects of:
• Insulin
• Oral hypoglycemia
Drugs That Increase Effect of Propranolol:
• Cimetidine
• Molindone
Drugs That Decrease the Effect of Propranolol:
• Carbamazepine
• Estrogens (birth control pills)
• Nicotine
• Nonsteroidal anti-inflammatory analgesics
When Used Together, Shared Inhibition of Propranolol and:
• Aminophylline
• Narcotic analgesics
• Sympathomimetics
• Theophylline

per minute, the next dose of propranolol should be withheld.
Decreasing subsequent doses of propranolol may be required.
An ECG should be performed. If an abnormality is documented
or if the vital signs do not return to normal, consultation with a
cardiologist is advisable. If a child develops an asthmatic
condition while on propranolol, the medication must be
discontinued immediately and the asthma treated

Table 11.13

**Dosage and Regimen of Propranolol for Pediatric
Psychiatry Patients**

Adolescents:
• No firm guidelines have been established
• Since used to treat many medical conditions, guidelines extrapolated to psychiatric patients
• Dose range 20–200 mg/day
• Start with dose 10 mg b.i.d.
• Increase by 10–20 mg every three to four days
Prepubertal Children:
• No firm guidelines have been established
• Dose range 10–120 mg/day
• Start with dose 10 mg per day
• Increase by 10 mg every three to four days

appropriately. The propranolol should *not* be reinstituted once
the asthma attack subsides. The hypoglycemic effects of
propranolol usually do not require intervention in nondiabetic
patients. Propranolol must be avoided if a patient is diabetic
since it may block symptoms of hypoglycemia in insulin
dependent patients. Determine whether there is a personal or
family history of depression prior to initiating propranolol
therapy and avoid using propranolol in such patients. When
depressive side effects are observed during propranolol therapy
in a patient who has shown favorable improvement in the
targeted condition, switching to atenolol should be considered,
as this medication is less commonly associated with depression.

Overdose

See Table 11.14.

An overdose of propranolol or other beta-blockers can have a
very high potential for causing death and is considered a
life-threatening emergency.

Abuse

Propranolol and the other beta-blockers have a very low risk of
abuse.

Table 11.14

Propranolol Overdose

Signs and Symptoms:

- Bradycardia
- Hypotension
- Cardiac arrest
- Respiratory distress
- GI symptoms, such as nausea and diarrhea
- Peripheral cyanosis
- Psychosis
- Seizures

Treatment of Overdose:

- Not dialyzable
- Immediate evacuation of gastric contents required
- For bradycardia, administer atropine 0.25–1.0 mg
- If no response, cautious administration of isoproterenol is recommended
- For hypotension, vasopressors, such as epinephrine, are indicated
- For cardiac failure, digitization and diuretics are necessary
- For bronchospasm, administer isoproterenol and aminophylline

---

References

1. Hunt, R.D., Capper, L., O'Connell, P. (1990). Clonidine in child and adolescent psychiatry. *J Child Adolesc Psychopharmacol, 1,* 87–101.
2. Leckman, J.F., Walkup, J.T., Cohen, D.J. (1988). Clonidine treatment of Tourette's syndrome. In D.J. Cohen, R.D. Bruun, J.F. Leckman (Eds.), *Tourette's Syndrome and Tic Disorders: Clinical Understanding and Treatment.* New York: Wiley.
3. Leckman, J.F., Detlor, J., Harcherik, D.F., et al. (1985). Short- and long-term treatment of Tourette's syndrome with clonidine: A clinical perspective. *Neurology, 35,* 343–351.
4. Leckman, J.F., Cohen, D.J., Detlor, J., et al. (1982). Clonidine in the treatment of Tourette's syndrome: A review of data. In A.J. Friedhoff, T.N. Chase (Eds.), *Gilles de la Tourette Syndrome* (pp. 391–401). New York: Raven Press.
5. Leckman, J.F., Cohen, D.J. (1983). Recent advances in Gilles de la Tourette's syndrome: Implications for clinical practice and future research. *Psychiatr Dev, 1,* 301–306.
6. Singer, H.S., Gammon, K., Quaskey, S. (1986). Haloperidol, fluphenazine, and clonidine in Tourette's syndrome: Controversies in treatment. *Pediatr Neurol Sci., 12,* 71–74.

7. Cohen, D.J., Detlor, J., Young, J.G., et al. (1980). Clonidine ameliorates Gilles de la Tourette's syndrome. *Arch Gen Psychiatry*, *37*, 1350–1354.

8. Bond, W.S. (1986). Psychiatric indications for clonidine: The neuropharmacologic and clinical basis. *J Clin Psychopharmacol*, *6*, 81.

9. Mesulam, M.M., Peterson, R.C. (1987). Treatment of Gilles de la Tourette's syndrome: Eight-year practice based experience in a predominantly adult population. *Neurology*, *37*, 1828–1833.

10. Arana, G.W., Hyman, S.E. (Eds.) (1991). *Handbook of Psychiatric Drug Therapy* (2nd ed.) (pp. 177–180). Boston: Little Brown.

11. Hunt, R.D., Arnsten, A.F.T., Asbell, M.D. (1995). An open trial of guanfacine in the treatment of attention deficit hyperactivity disorder. *J Am Acad Child Adolesc Psychiatry*, *34*, 50–54.

12. Chappell, P.B., Riddle, M.A., Scahill, L., et al. (1995). Guanfacine treatment of comorbid attention deficit hyperactivity disorder and Tourette's syndrome: Preliminary clinical experience. *J Am Acad Child Adolesc Psychiatry*. *34*, 1147–1152.

13. Horrigan, J.P., Barnhill, L.J. (1995). Guanfacine and treatment-resistant attention-deficit hyperactivity disorder in boys. *J Child Adolesc Psychopharmacol*, *5*, 215–224.

Opiate Antagonists

Opiate antagonists play a limited but potentially useful role in child psychiatry. Naltrexone (Trexan) and the older drug, naloxone, were originally produced to study and treat opiate toxicity (see Chapter 14). However, naltrexone was available in tablet form and soon found other uses.

Indications

Self-Injurious Behavior

Self-injurious behavior (SIB) is a common symptom of psychiatric illness, especially in children with severe developmental disability. It has been suggested that children who chronically self-abuse may be less sensitive to pain owing to their increased levels of endogenous opioids. In fact, naltrexone does appear to decrease SIB in placebo-controlled studies, at doses of 0.5 to 1.5 mg/kg/day.[1–3] Doses outside of this range are less effective. Although more study is needed, the authors have found naltrexone to be a useful tool for a subset of children who self-abuse, especially when used in conjunction with an aggressive behavioral modification program. Naltrexone alone without behavioral therapy often leads to relapse.

See Table 12.1.

Autistic Disorder

Autistic children often exhibit SIB, but also have other characteristics that have been loosely compared to opiate intoxication (social withdrawal, stereotypy, and sensory hyper- or hyposensitivity). A few small, but well-done, studies have reported improvement of these autistic symptoms on

Table 12.1

Possible Indications for Opiate Antagonists

Self-injurious behavior	Recommended
Autistic disorder	Recommended
Obesity	Not recommended
Eating disorders	Not recommended

naltrexone.[4,5] Given the lack of other available treatments and the low risks associated with naltrexone, we consider this a reasonable treatment option for children with autism, if they exhibit the symptoms noted above. The optimal dose is uncertain, but is likely between 0.5 and 2.0 mg/kg/day.

Obesity and Eating Disorders

Naltrexone has received some attention as a possible treatment for anorexia, bulimia, and obesity, largely based on animal studies. However, controlled studies on humans do not support the effectiveness of naltrexone for these disorders.

Contraindications

Elevated hepatic enzymes may appear at very high doses. Therefore, naltrexone should not be used when there is preexisting hepatic disease. The only additional contraindications relate to the concurrent use of, withdrawal from, or dependence on opiate drugs, since naltrexone may cause precipitous opiate withdrawal in such cases.

Side Effects

In the studies cited, mild sedation was the only reported adverse effect in children. Insomnia, anxiety, and GI upset are listed as infrequent side effects, but have not been reported in clinical studies. There are no reported cases of overdose.

Initiating and Maintaining Treatment

Baseline and periodic liver function studies are recommended and the drug should be discontinued in the unlikely event of hepatic toxicity. Some children will respond to a low dose of

0.5 mg/kg/day. Since even lower doses have not been tested, clinical use should start at 0.25 mg/kg/day in a single dose, with gradual increases every one to two weeks. The 50-mg scored tablet may be quartered or crushed to allow for fine increments. The average dose found effective in studies is 1.5 mg/kg/day. A dose of 2.0 mg/kg/day should be considered the maximum, since no studies have reported improvement at higher doses.

References

1. Barrett, R.P., Feinstein, C., Hole, W.T. (1989). Effects of naloxone and naltrexone on self-injury: A double-blind, placebo-controlled analysis. *Am J Ment Retard*, *93*, 644–651.
2. Herman, B.H., Hammock, M.K., Arthur-Smith, A., et al. (1987). Naltrexone decreases self-injurious behavior. *Ann Neurol*, *22*, 550–552.
3. Sandman, C.A., Barron, J.L., Colman, H. (1990). An orally administered opiate blocker, naltrexone, attenuates self-injurious behavior. *Am J Ment Retard*, *95*, 93–102.
4. Leboyer, M., Bouvard, M.P., Launay, J.M., et al. (1992). Brief report: A double-blind study of naltrexone in infantile autism. *J Autism Dev Disord*, *22*, 309–319.
5. Panksepp, J., Lensing, P. (1991). Brief report: A synopsis of an open-trial of naltrexone treatment of autism with four children. *J Autism Dev Disord*, *21*, 243–249.

Consultation–Liaison Psychiatry—Pharmacologic Approaches

We believe the following areas to be especially relevant to the child and adolescent psychiatrist in the medical and surgical setting: (1) psychiatric consultation to neurology, (2) psychiatric consultation to pediatrics, and (3) psychiatric consultation to obstetrics and gynecology.

Psychiatric Consultation to Neurology

Epilepsy, one of the most common chronic illnesses of childhood, has a very high prevalence of associated psychiatric dysfunction.[1] Patients with other neurologic disorders necessitating psychiatric consultation include those who, after brain trauma, develop aggressive, disruptive, and/or depressed behavior. Some patients have exacerbations or recurrences of psychiatric symptoms.[2] It may be difficult to determine whether the condition is attributable to an emotional reaction, is caused by neurologic disability, is due to the neurologic pathology, or results from a combination of all three. For patients in whom neurologic and physical examination fails to find an organic basis for the symptoms, the psychiatrist may be called on to determine whether there is a psychogenic cause, that is, a somatization disorder, conversion disorder, or the like.[2]

Table 13.1

Personality Profile of Temporal Lobe Epilepsy Patients

Behaviors	**Thought**	**Mood**
• Obsessionalism • Circumstantiality • Hypergraphia • Dependence	• Philosophical • Religious • Humorlessness	• Mood swings • Anger • Sadness

From Bear, D.M., Fedio, P. (1977). Quantitative analysis of interictal behavior in temporal lobe epilepsy. *Arch Neurol, 34,* 454–467.

Epilepsy

The rate of psychiatric disorder has been found to be higher among epileptic children than in healthy controls or in children with other chronic illnesses. It also appears that epileptic patients have a distinctive personality profile, such that those with temporal lobe epilepsy (TLE) have distinctive features of behavior, emotion, and thought (Table 13.1).

Organic Personality Disorder

Organic personality disorder occurs in 20% of TLE patients. Predictors of the development of organic personality disorder are an early age of onset of epilepsy and protracted course of the illness.[3]

See Table 13.1.

Mood Disorders and Suicide

Bipolar disorder symptoms are associated with right hemisphere TLE and with about 30% of epileptics' attempting suicide. The suicide rate for epileptics is about four times that of the general population.[4] Epileptic attempters made more medically serious attempts, had more premeditation prior to the attempts and had a higher suicide intent before and after the attempts than did nonepileptic attempters. There is a growing concern that part of the psychiatric morbidity in childhood epilepsy may be attributable to the effects of antiepileptic medications.[5]

Phenobarbital-Induced Psychiatric Dysfunction

Patients treated with phenobarbital as compared with carbamazepine showed a significantly higher prevalence of major depressive disorder (40% versus 4%) and suicidal ideation (47% versus 4%), with the higher prevalence in patients with a family history of mood disorder among first-degree relatives. An alternative treatment (i.e., carbamazepine) was advocated for patients with newly diagnosed epilepsy and a personal or family history of mood disorder.

Phenobarbital has been associated with an increased risk of psychological disturbances in addition to depression and suicidal ideation, including hyperactivity, irritability, sleep difficulties, poor self-esteem, mood fluctuations, neurotic symptoms, and conduct problems.[6]

Panic Attacks

Epileptic patients may have panic attacks that often prove difficult to delineate from the primary seizure disorder.[7] Consultation with a neurologist is indicated. In patients determined to have a seizure disorder in addition to panic attacks, stabilization of seizures with anticonvulsants is recommended with subsequent standard anti-panic treatment. It should be noted that benzodiazepines which can be effective in panic attacks can also be helpful in treating seizures.

Psychosis

Psychosis is often associated with TLE. Antipsychotic medication may be warranted to treat such patients.

Seizures That are Uncontrolled

A psychogenic etiology may need to be considered, and this often is not an all-or-none phenomenon. In addition, stress can exacerbate or induce genuine seizures in vulnerable patients. Sleep deprivation has been associated with increased seizures. These various types of seizures can often be differentiated on clinical criteria, along with 24-hour video and EEG monitoring.

Psychiatric Effects of Anticonvulsants

Anticonvulsants are discussed in Chapter 9. Polydrug therapy is associated with more adverse neuropsychiatric and behavioral side effects than is monodrug therapy.[8] Benzodiazepines can produce behavioral disinhibition, leading to increased irritability and aggression. Phenytoin and phenobarbital appear to have more pronounced behavioral effects than carbamazepine or valproic acid. Many of these side effects are reversible. Cognitive impairment has been observed on chronic treatment with phenytoin and/or phenobarbital.[9]

Antipsychotics and antidepressants have been reported to lower the seizure threshold. Bupropion, a nonheterocyclic antidepressant, should probably be avoided in epileptic and brain-damaged patients because of an increased incidence of seizures (see Chapter 4).

Psychotic and aggressive patients who present a clear danger to themselves and/or others may require antipsychotic intervention. If a child is on an effective anticonvulsant regimen, antipsychotics can be cautiously introduced. Molindone and fluphenazine have been shown to have the lowest potential for decreasing the seizure threshold.[10]

Metabolic Diseases of the Nervous System

Phenylketonuria

The majority of phenylketonuria patients are severely mentally retarded. Hyperactivity and erratic and unpredictable behavior are frequently observed.[11] They can be difficult to manage and exhibit a variety of behaviors, including bizarre movements of their extremities, and may resemble autistic or schizophrenic patients. They may have many perceptual difficulties, have difficulty with communication, and appear to be uncoordinated. Convulsions are present in approximately one third of all cases. It is always important to investigate the medications the patient is currently receiving and to assess their risk of contributing to the problem behaviors.

Wilson's Disease

Wilson's disease is an autosomal recessive disorder that results in liver dysfunction, jaundice, and Kayser-Fleischer rings in the cornea. Psychiatric symptoms are often prominent; may precede medical and neurologic signs; and include irritability, depression, psychosis, and hepatic encephalopathy with profound mental changes. Mood swings are common and can be explosive. Patients may become combative and symptoms sometimes resemble those of schizophrenia. Memory loss may occur, and may be particularly upsetting to the patient. Pharmacologic intervention may be necessary.

Lesch-Nyhan Syndrome

This is a disorder of purine metabolism and is characterized by hyperuricemia associated with spasticity and severe choreoathetosis. These patients often self-mutilate, such as by involuntarily biting their fingers, arms, and lips, or pulling out clumps of their hair. Physical restraint is often required. Pharmacologic intervention, including neuroleptics, is frequently necessary. Various agents have been found anecdotally to be helpful in the treatment of SIB (see Chapters 8, 9, 11, and 12).

Psychopharmacologic Treatment of Psychiatric Sequelae of Neurologic Disease

Neurologically impaired patients are more sensitive to the side effects of psychotropic medications. It is best to begin with a low dose and increase it slowly over longer periods.[2]

Depression

Depression may warrant a trial of the newer antidepressants (see Chapter 5).

Mania

Mania associated with head trauma/injury and other CNS lesions has, in adults, been successfully treated with lithium, carbamazepine, valproic acid, and electroconvulsive therapy (ECT).[12] These treatments can exacerbate confusion and induce mental-status changes in patients with CNS impairment. Similar treatment principles, such as administering the medication in small divided doses (see Chapter 7) and increasing gradually while monitoring for side effects, apply to children and adolescents. We advocate the use of carbamazepine in the treatment of mania and epilepsy, since this allows monodrug therapy.

Psychosis

Psychotic children and adolescents with neurologic disorders should be treated with antipsychotic medications when their behavior can be dangerous to themselves or others (see Chapter 7). An acute dystonic reaction is easily treatable with diphenhydramine or benztropine mesylate. Neuroleptics should be avoided in the acute phases of recovery after brain injury.[13] We recommend low-dose haloperidol, 0.5 mg b.i.d., or fluphenazine, 0.5 mg b.i.d.[13]

Anxiety

For acute panic attacks, low-dose benzodiazepines may be required for short-term use. Buspirone may be tried as it has a favorable side-effects profile and is not addictive (see Chapter 10). SSRIs and TCAs are generally not helpful for acute panic attacks, but can be effective in their long-term treatment.

Psychiatric Consultation to Pediatrics

Endocrine Disorders

Diabetes

Pharmacologic intervention is a last resort for these patients. Mental status changes (delirium, anxiety, irritability, etc.) often resolve once the underlying medical disturbance is corrected. If psychiatric symptoms persist, psychotic patients can be treated with low-dose neuroleptics. If depression persists, treatment with the newer antidepressants may be considered (see Chapter 5).

Thyroid Disease

Hypothyroidism   In adults, hypothyroidism may present with apathy or depressive symptoms without accompanying physical symptoms. The prevalence is believed to be lower in children and adolescents. Screening, including thyroid function tests and especially TSH, is performed on young people with unexplained psychiatric symptoms. One should first treat the underlying condition (with thyroid replacement therapy), then monitor to determine whether the psychiatric symptoms persist after thyroid replacement therapy. Antidepressants may be considered in depression refractory to non-pharmacologic interventions, with short-term benzodiazepine use indicated for acute anxiety and/or panic states. For a discussion of lithium-induced hypothyroidism, see Chapter 8.

Hyperthyroidism   If psychosocial and behavioral interventions prove unsuccessful, psychopharmacologic management may be indicated. Although TCAs are contraindicated for children and adolescents with hyperthyroidism and depression because of the risk of cardiac arrhythmias,[14] a trial of the new antidepressants may be warranted (see Chapter 5). Benzodiazepines or beta-blockers may be warranted in patients with significant anxiety.

Gastrointestinal Disorders

Irritable Bowel Syndrome
These patients have a high frequency of depression. Anxiolytics and antidepressants also have been used in the treatment of irritable bowel syndrome.[15]

Inflammatory Bowel Disease
A high frequency of depression in patients with inflammatory bowel disease has been reported. We recommend an approach similar to that advocated in the other sections of this chapter. The TCAs should be avoided because of their anticholinergic effects, which may exacerbate the underlying medical condition.

Connective Tissue Disease

Systemic Lupus Erythematosus
Patients with systemic lupus erythematosus (SLE) are particularly vulnerable to delirium because of multisystem involvement.[16] Delirium induced by steroids is not uncommonly seen in SLE patients, since high doses of steroids are often used to treat disease exacerbations. The treatment of choice for steroid-induced delirium is first to lower the steroid to the lowest possible effective dose, and then, when necessary, to use a low-dose neuroleptic, such as haloperidol, 1 to 2 mg/day. The neuroleptic should only be required for acute psychosis and discontinued as soon as possible.[16]

Renal Disease

Patients with renal failure who require dialysis and/or are awaiting kidney transplant not uncommonly exhibit neuropsychiatric symptoms (depression, anxiety, psychosis, delirium, cognitive impairment) that merit psychiatric consultation.[16]

Pharmacologic Considerations in Renal Failure
Lithium is the main psychotropic whose drug levels are primarily dependent on renal clearance mechanisms (see Chapter 8). To avoid some of the difficulties with lithium in treating mania, alternative antimanic agents, such as carbamazepine or valproic acid, may be considered.

See Table 13.2.

Table 13.2

Psychiatric Side Effects of Cardiac Drugs

Tocainide, Mexiletin, Lidocaine	Flecainide	Amiodarone	Captopril, Enalapril, Lisinopril	Digitalis
Anxiety Psychosis Dizziness Agitation	Anxiety or dizziness	Depression, confusion	Elevation or depression of mood	Illusions Depression Delirium

Table 13.3

Bronchodilator Drug Interactions

Theophylline:
- Increases renal clearance of lithium
- May cause anxiety, jitteriness, nervousness when combined with CNS stimulants

Psychotropic Drugs and Asthma

Stress can induce or exacerbate an asthmatic attack. In some cases, children who have had life-threatening asthma attacks necessitating intubation and who require frequent hospitalizations may experience chronic anxiety and/or panic attacks. Benzodiazepines can depress ventilation and be life-threatening for asthmatic patients, particularly in the midst of an acute exacerbation. These agents should be avoided.

Buspirone may be safer than benzodiazepines in the treatment of anxiety in children and adolescents with asthma. It may be tried for chronically anxious asthmatic children and adolescents, particularly where the anxiety is interfering with treatment, starting with a low test dose of 10 mg/day and increasing it gradually by 10-mg increments every five to seven days to a maximum of 40 mg/day.

Nonselective beta-blockers, such as propranolol, are absolutely contraindicated for patients with asthma.

See Tables 13.3 through 13.11.

Table 13.4

Side Effects of Theophylline

- Anxiety
- Mental status changes and seizures
- Depression
- ADHD—unproven
- Learning disabilities—unproven

Table 13.5

Neuropsychiatric Side Effects of Albuterol

- Anxiety
- Psychosis
- Mania
- Antidepressant—unproven

Table 13.6

Aerosol–Inhaler–Induced Psychiatric Side Effects

- Psychological addiction
- Anxiety
- Agitation
- Disorientation
- Greater risk of toxicity to children

AIDS

In children, the most common manifestation of the acquired immunodeficiency syndrome (AIDS) is failure to thrive, with loss of developmental milestones.[17] The human immunodeficiency virus (HIV) can directly infect CNS cells, and can cause encephalopathy, motor dysfunction, meningitis, seizures, and cerebral tumors. Children can also experience profound neuropsychological impairment characterized by a gross deterioration in cognitive functioning.[18] Neurovegetative symptoms of depression, including apathy and psychomotor

Table 13.7

**Psychiatric Side Effects
of Decongestants**

Ephedrine
- Anxiety
- Dysphoria
- Irritability
- Restlessness
- Insomnia
- Psychosis
- Mania

Phenylpropanolamine
- Psychosis
- Agitation and restlessness
- Irritability
- Aggressiveness
- Organic brain syndromes
- Children especially vulnerable

Naphazoline
- Sedation
- Coma

Table 13.8

Cautions When Using Decongestants

Use Decongestants with Caution
- When prescribing CNS psychostimulants a potentiation of side effects is possible
- Be alert for psychosis and mania
- Avoid phenylpropanolamine for children and adolescents
- Phenylpropanolamine absolutely contraindicated if patient is receiving MAOI
- Naphazoline contraindicated in children less than 6 years old

---

Table 13.9

**Psychiatric Side Effects of
Anticholinergic Agents**

Central Anticholinergic Syndrome
- Peripheral muscarinic blockade
- Acute psychosis
- Ataxia
- Myotonic twitching
- Increased muscle tone and muscular weakening
- Toxic delirium
- Impaired GI motility (paralytic ileus)

Table 13.10

**Side Effects of
Expectorant
Mucolytic Agents**

- Goiter/hypothyroidism
- Nervousness
- Insomnia

Table 13.11

**Psychiatric Side Effects of
Central Cough Suppressants**

Codeine
- Agitation
- Combative behavior
- Sedation

Dextromethorphan
- Excitation
- Confusion
- Opiate-like respiratory depression
- Hypomania

retardation, can also be presenting symptoms of children infected with the AIDS virus.

Organic brain syndromes caused by HIV infection of the brain can mimic psychiatric disorders, such as major depression, suicide, psychosis, mania, OCD, and dementia. Pharmacotherapy is generally an intervention of last resort.

Pharmacotherapy in Children and Adolescents with AIDS
Depression   Serotonin reuptake inhibitors, such as fluoxetine and sertraline, and other available antidepressants, such as bupropion, venlafaxine, and trazodone, that have no anticholinergic side effects may be more appropriate for these patients. Bupropion has a higher risk of seizure than many other antidepressants. Trazodone can be quite sedating and may have orthostatic side effects. It should be emphasized that there has been no systematic study of the use of any of the aforementioned agents for children and adolescents with AIDS.

Psychosis   Severe psychosis with danger to the patient or others may require pharmacologic intervention. A high-potency neuroleptic, such as haloperidol or risperidone, is preferred to low-potency agents, such as thioridazine and chlorpromazine, which have more anticholinergic side effects, since the former is less likely to exacerbate an organic mental syndrome.

Agitation / Aggression   Low-dose haloperidol or risperidone may also be indicated for patients with severe agitation (not necessarily due to psychosis). AIDS patients who are having acute anxiety and/or panic attacks may require short-term benzodiazepine intervention, particularly if the anxiety is compromising the patient's medical/respiratory status. Low-dose lorazepam may be of value with doses of 1 to 2 mg as needed for acute attacks. Careful monitoring of the patient's mental status is essential. The non-benzodiazepine anxiolytic buspirone may also be considered in these cases. It can be started at a dose of 10 mg b.i.d. to t.i.d. It frequently takes two to four weeks to exert a full effect (see Chapter 10).

Mania   In the event that an HIV-infected patient becomes manic, treatment with lithium may be warranted. Extreme caution is required when using lithium for AIDS patients as they will be sensitive to its neurologic side effects (see Chapter 8). Carbamazepine or valproic acid may be tried.

Psychiatric Consultation to Oncology

The association of psychiatric disorders with cancer has been well documented, most commonly depression. Many of the chemotherapy regimens can cause psychiatric complications.

Pharmacologic Interventions in Children and Adolescents with Cancer

Neuroleptics
Medically ill patients may be more susceptible to neuroleptic side effects, especially neuroleptic malignant syndrome (NMS).[19] In cancer patients, it is advisable to keep neuroleptic doses low by adding benzodiazepines for the management of agitation.[19] Lorazepam is the benzodiazepines of choice. Metoclopramide, which is frequently used as an antiemetic during chemotherapy, requires close monitoring for adverse effects, especially extrapyrimidal syndrome (EPS).[19]

Patients with significant depression may be tried on such agents as SSRIs or the newer antidepressants (see Chapter 5).

Pain Management

See Table 13.12.

Opioids: Administration
Opioids are the primary agents utilized in the treatment of chronic cancer pain.[20] Opioids can be administered orally, IV, subcutaneously, IM, transdermally, transmucosally, or directly into the epidural and subarachnoid space.[21] They can produce sedation, respiratory depression, GI intolerance, cough suppression, and vasodilation.[22] Administration of sedative hypnotics with opioids can significantly increase the sedative and respiratory depressant effects of opioids.

See Tables 13.13 and 13.14.

Stimulants
Methylphenidate and dextroamphetamine have been shown to decrease narcotic requirements and narcotic-induced CNS depression.[22]

See Table 13.15.

Table 13.12

Nonopioid Peripherally Acting Analgesics

Acetaminophen
- Most common analgesic for children and adolescents in the United States
- First medication used in mild to moderate pain
- Combination with codeine (Tylenol 3) treats severe pain
- High therapeutic ratio
- Give in doses 10–20 mg/kg every four hours
- Does not cause gastritis and bleeding
- Neuropathy and liver damage unlikely at therapeutic doses

Salicylates
- Associated with Reye's syndrome
- Can cause gastritis and platelet dysfunction
- Should not be used in pediatric population

Non-Steroidal Anti-Inflammatory Drugs (NSAIDs)
- Minimal study in children
- Give with food to decrease GI upset
- Relieve pain by inhibiting prostaglandin synthesis
- Concern about bleeding problem in children

Table 13.13

Opiate Agonists and Antagonists

Pure opiate agonists
- Include morphine, methadone, fentanyl
- No ceiling effect
- Increased dose results in increased pain relief

Mixed agonist–antagonists
- Include pentazocine, butorphanol, propoxyphene
- Have ceiling effect
- Can antagonize and reverse actions of pure agonists
- Associated with high rate of dysphoria
- May precipitate opiate withdrawal

Opiate antagonists
- Include naloxone, naltrexone
- Reverse opiate-induced analgesia, sedation, and respiratory depression
- Chronic administration can result in anxiety, depression, nausea, vomiting, and pulmonary edema

Table 13.14

Specific Opioids

Morphine
- Effective in ameliorating pediatric pain
- In opioid-naïve patients, starting doses are 0.1 mg/kg IV every two hours, or 0.1 mg/kg IM or SQ every three to four hours
- Acute oral-to-parenteral ratio 6 : 1
- Chronic oral-to-parenteral ratio 3 : 1
- Time-release oral preparations of morphine allow b.i.d. or t.i.d. dosing
- Need to monitor neuropsychiatric function

Codeine
- Most commonly administered oral opioid for moderate pain
- Starting dose 0.5 mg/kg PO every four hours

Methadone
- Longer duration of action than morphine or heroin
- Metabolized very slowly
- Unlike heroin, can be given orally
- Somnolence relatively common and necessitates dosage reduction
- In children, oral administration of methadone every six to eight hours or IV every four to six hours following a loading dose yields consistent clinical effect
- Initial oral doses: 0.1 mg/kg every four hours, and then every six to eight hours

Fentanyl
- Much shorter duration of action after bolus administration than morphine
- Useful when analgesia is required for brief but painful procedures
- Doses for painful procedures: 102 μg/kg or increasing dose by 0.5 μg/kg every 1–2 minutes p.r.n.

Meperidine (Demerol)
- Shorter duration of action than morphine
- Active metabolite normeperidine associated with convulsions and dysphoria

Hydromorphone (Dilaudid)
- Eight times more potent than morphine
- Oral-to-parenteral ratio 3–4 : 1
- Oral preparation better tolerated than oral morphine preparation

---

Table 13.15

Naloxone Administration

- Used in emergency treatment of opioid overdose
- Doses of 0.01–0.02 mg/kg cause complete reversal of opiate agonist effects
- When possible, give lower dose of 0.002 mg/kg to attenuate respiratory depression without completely reversing sedative and analgesic effects
- Duration of action 30–45 minutes
- Monitor closely for relapse respiratory depression

References

1. Hauser, W., Kurland, L. (1975). The epidemiology of epilepsy in Rochester, Minnesota: 1935 through 1967. *Epilepsia, 16*, 1–66.
2. Hales, R.E., Thompson, T.L. (1991). Consultation–liaison psychiatry. In A. Tasman, S.M. Goldfinger, C.A. Kaufmann (Eds.), *Review of Psychiatry* (vol. 9) (pp. 433–566). Washington, DC: American Psychiatric Press.
3. Garyfallos, G., Manos, N., Adamopoulou, A. (1988). Psychopathology and personality characteristics of epileptic patients: Epilepsy, psychopathology and personality. *Acta Psychiatr Scand, 78*, 87–95.
4. Brent, D.A. (1986). Overrepresentation of epileptics in a consecutive series of suicide attempters seen at Children's Hospital, 1978–1983. *J Am Acad Child Psychiatry, 25*, 242–246.
5. American Academy of Pediatrics, Committee on Drugs. (1985). Behavioral and cognitive effects of anticonvulsant therapy. *Pediatrics, 76*, 644–647.
6. Brent, D.A., Crumrine, P.K., Varma, R.R., et al. (1987). Phenobarbital treatment and major depressive disorder in children with epilepsy. *Pediatrics, 80*, 909–917.
7. Weilberg, J.B., Bear, D.M., Sachs, G. (1989). Three patients with concomitant panic attacks and seizure disorder: Possible clues to the neurology of anti-anxiety. *Am J Psychiatry, 144*, 1053–1056.
8. Hoare, P. (1984). The development of psychiatric disorder among school children with epilepsy. *Dev Med Child Neurol, 26*, 3–13.
9. Corbett, J.A., Trimble, M.R., Nichol, T.C. (1985). Behavioral and cognitive impairments in children with epilepsy: The long-term effects of anticonvulsant therapy. *J Am Acad Child Psychiatry, 24*, 17–23.
10. Oliver, A.P., Luchins, D.J., Wyatt, R.J. (1982). Neuroleptic-induced seizures: An in vitro technique for assessing relative risk. *Arch Gen Psychiatry, 39*, 206–209.
11. Menkes, J.H. (1990). Tumors of the nervous system. In J.H. Menkes (Ed.), *Textbook of Child Neurology* (4th ed.) (pp. 526–582). Philadelphia: Lea & Febiger.

12. Stewart, J.T., Nemsath, R.H. (1988). Bipolar illness following traumatic brain injury: Treatment with lithium and carbamazepine. *J Clin Psychiatry, 49,* 74–75.

13. Silver, J.M., Hales, R.E., Yudofsky, S.C. (1990). Psychiatric consultation to neurology. In A. Tasman, S.M. Goldfinger, C.A. Kaufmann (Eds.), *Review of Psychiatry* (vol. 9) (pp. 433–465). Washington, DC: American Psychiatric Press.

14. Blackwell, B., Schmidt, G.L. (1984). Drug interactions in psychopharmacology. *Psychiatr Clin North Am, 7,* 625–636.

15. Rhodes, J.B., Abrams, H.J., Manning, R.T. (1978). Controlled clinical trial of sedative-anticholinergic drugs in patients with irritable bowel syndrome. *J Clin Pharmacal, 18,* 340–345.

16. Stoudemire, G.A., Levenson, J.L. (1991). Psychiatric consultation to internal medicine. In A. Tasman, S.M. Goldfinger, C.A. Kaufmann (Eds.), *Review of Psychiatry* (vol. 9) (pp. 460–490). Washington, DC: American Psychiatric Press.

17. Belfer, M.L., Munir, K. (1991). Acquired immunodeficiency syndrome. In J.M. Wiener (Ed.), *Textbook of Child and Adolescent Psychiatry* (1st ed.) (pp. 495–506). Washington, DC: American Psychiatric Press.

18. Belman, A.L., Diamond, G., Dickson, D., et al. (1988). Pediatric acquired immunodeficiency syndrome: Neurologic syndromes. *Am J Dis Child, 149,* 29–35.

19. Lederberg, M.S., Massie, M.J., Hollard, J.C. (1991). Psychiatric consultation to oncology. In A. Tasman, S.M. Goldfinger, C.A. Kaufmann (Eds.), *Review of Psychiatry* (vol. 9) (pp. 491–514). Washington, DC: American Psychiatric Press.

20. Foley, K.M. (1979). Pain syndromes in patients with cancer. *Adv Pain Res Ther, 2,* 59–75.

21. Payne, R. (1987). *Principles of Analgesic Use in the Treatment of Acute Pain and Chronic Cancer Pain.* Washington, DC: American Pain Society.

22. Shannon, M., Berde, C.B. (1989). Pharmacologic management of pain in children and adolescents. *Pediatr Clin North Am, 36,* 855–870.

C h a p t e r   14

Treatment of Substance Abuse Disorders

The major controversy regarding the psychopharmacologic management of substance abuse disorders has centered on whether such an approach is indicated at all for these patients. Uncontrolled studies on adults have shown that healthy patients in drug or alcohol withdrawal can be treated safely and successfully without using psychotropic medications. Some front-line nonphysician clinicians are adamantly opposed to the use of psychotropic medications for patients who have preexisting substance abuse disorders. Recent studies of the biological and genetic basis of inherited forms of substance abuse disorders have heightened interest in potential psychopharmacologic interventions. *There have been, as yet, almost no studies of these treatments for children or adolescents with substance abuse disorders. Thus, recommendations for the treatment of children and adolescents are based on extrapolations from adults—an approach with obvious limitations and potential hazards.*

Potential Differences Between Adolescent and Adult Substance Abuse Disorder

- Adolescents may have increased vulnerability to substance abuse and/or dependence.
- Adolescents may engage in more polydrug abuse.
- Adolescents may *not* experience the life-threatening side effects of withdrawal from alcohol that adults experience.

Table 14.1

Epidemiology of Alcohol and Drug Use in High School Seniors, College Students, and Young Adults

	Ever Used	Frequent Use/Abuse	Notes
Alcohol[1]	90%	3.7% daily use	Alcohol and tobacco may be "gateway drugs" leading to subsequent use of other substances
Nicotine[1]	66%	33% with daily use 10% smoke one-half pack per day or more	Very low (20%) rate of noncontinuation of daily smokers
Marijuana[2]	41%	14% some use within past one month 2% daily use	
Cocaine[3]	9%		44% noncontinuation rate of users
Crack cocaine	3.5%		46% noncontinuation rate
Inhalants and amyl and butyl nitrites	2%	0.3% daily use	More frequent use in males than females
Hallucinogens	2.8% for phencyclidine (PCP) 8.7% for LSD	0.3% daily use of hallucinogens	
Opiates	8% for opiates other than heroi 1.3% heroin		High noncontinuation rates
Sedatives	2.3% for methaqualone 6.8% for barbiturates		50% noncontinuation rate

Table 14.2

Definitions: Intoxication, Tolerance, and Dependence

Intoxication	Disturbance of normal CNS function caused by the pharmacologic characteristics of the drug
Tolerance	Change that occurs in an individual as a result of repeated exposure to a drug so that less effect is produced by taking the same amount of the drug and an increased amount is required to produce the same effect
Dependence	Use of substance leading to significant impairment in the person's functioning in which tolerance, withdrawal, and continued use of the substance despite adverse consequences. (DSM-IV-R)

Table 14.3

Treatment Strategies (All Data from Adult Studies)

Opiates
Withdrawal

Methadone, a long-acting opiate with a half-life of 15–22 hours, substitutes for other opiate; doses are titrated to target withdrawal symptoms; after maintaining the patient symptom-free for 24 hours, gradual reduction (e.g., 10–20% per day) is begun. *There are no data on children or adolescents and many practitioners are hesitant to prescribe this additive drug (methadone) for children.* Clonidine is given in oral daily doses of 1–2 mg (in adults) to treat withdrawal symptoms. It may be combined with naltrexone, which will precipitate rapid withdrawal that may then be managed with clonidine.

Treatment

Methadone in sufficient doses blocks the effects of street drug opiates and attenuates drug-seeking activity and resultant criminal activity.
Naltrexone (a pure opiate antagonist).

Alcohol
Withdrawal

Withdrawal symptoms in adolescents are rare so pharmacologic treatment frequently is not needed. Diazepam (Valium)[4] loading with oral doses of 20 mg every two hours (for adults) until the patient is asymptomatic, then given as needed to prevent withdrawal symptoms.

(Continued)

Table 14.3

(Continued)

Clonidine[5] may be used to treat withdrawal symptoms but it does not have anticonvulsant effects. More study is needed.

Treatment

Lithium carbonate treatment decreases intoxication and cognitive and psychomotor performance deficits when challenged with alcohol and decrease the desire to continue drinking in one study, but another study found no effect of lithium on the course of alcoholism. More study is needed.

Naltrexone[6] 50 mg/day in adult male alcoholics resulted in less craving, fewer days of alcohol consumption, and a lower rate of relapse.

Disulfiram[7]—use of alcohol while on disulfiram results in highly aversive acetaldehyde reaction. Not better than placebo in one study. Significant potential toxicities result in this agent's not being recommended in children and adolescents. Specific SSRIs attenuate alcohol consumption independent of their effects on depression. Bromocriptine and apomorphine (dopamine agonists) may reduce alcohol craving but little controlled data are available to suggest their use.

Cocaine

Withdrawal

Bromocriptine, a dopamine receptor agonist, decreases cocaine craving. Buprenorphine. TCAs decreased cocaine craving in open studies, however, one controlled study showed no superiority over placebo.

Nicotine

Withdrawal

Nicotine-replacement therapy using polacrilex chewing gum (Nicorette) or nicotine transdermal system (Nicoderm, Prostep, Habitrol) may allow a successful slow taper. Transdermal systems were more effective than placebo in producing smoking cessation in double-blind studies. Dosing strategy is 21 mg for six weeks followed by 14 mg for two weeks, 7 mg for two weeks, then discontinuation.

Continued smoking while using nicotine-replacement therapy can result in nicotine poisoning. Because of the hazard of smoking (peer pressure) while using nicotine-replacement therapy we are not recommending this treatment for adolescents given the absence of data on this treatment for this population to date.

Risk Factors for Adolescent Substance Abuse

- Positive family history of substance abuse.
- Friends who use drugs.
- Physical and/or sexual abuse.
- Other (preexisting) psychiatric disorder, especially ADHD, conduct disorder, or depression.

See Tables 14.1, 14.2, and 14.3.

References

1. Johnston, L.D., O'Malley, P.M., Bachman, J.G. (1991). *U.S. Department of Health and Human Services: Drug Use Among American High School Seniors. College Students and Young Adults, 1975–1990*. Vol. 1 NIDA. DHHS Publication No. (ADM) 91-1813.
2. Marks, I., Lader, M. (1973). Anxiety states (anxiety neurosis): A review. *J Nerv Ment Dis, 156*, 3.
3. Shaffer, D., Fisher, P. (1981). The epidemiology of suicide in children and young adolescents. *J Am Acad Child Psychiatry, 20*, 545–565.
4. Sellers, E.M., Naranjo, C.A., Harrison, B., et al. (1983). Diazepam loading: Simplified treatment of alcohol withdrawal. *Clin Pharmacol Ther, 34*, 822–826.
5. Wilkins, A.J., Jenkins, W.J., Steiner, J.A. (1983). Efficacy of clonidine in the treatment of alcohol withdrawal state. *Psychopharmacology, 81*, 78–80.
6. Dole, U.P., Nyswander, M. (1965). A medical treatment for diacetylmorphine (heroin) addiction: A clinical trial with methadone hydrochloride. *JAMA, 193*, 646–650.
7. Fuller, R.K., Branchley, L., Brightivell, D.R., et al. (1986). Disulfiram treatment of alcoholism: A Veteran's Administration cooperative study. *JAMA, 256*, 1449–1455.

Index

A

Abnormal Involuntary Movement Scale (AIMS), and MAOI withdrawal, 76

Abuse
of anxiolytics/sedatives, 130–131
of beta-blockers, 153
of bupropion, 60
of clonidine, 145
of psychoactive drugs, neuroleptic treatment of, 80
of psychostimulants, 26, 26*t*
of tricyclic antidepressants, 41

Acquired immunodeficiency syndrome, 167–171

Acute depression, and lithium, 100

Acute dystonia, as antipsychotic side effect, 86–88

Acute lithium intoxication, 106*t*, 106–107

Acute mania, and lithium, 99–100

Adderall, and ADHD, 4–5, 24

ADHD
and anticonvulsants, 116
and antipsychotic agents, 82
and bupropion, 62*t*
and clonidine, 139, 144*t*
and guanfacine, 146

and lithium, 102
and MAOIs, 69
and psychostimulants, 12–26, 23*t*
recent developments in, 4–5
and SSRIs, 46, 56
and tic disorders (Tourette's Syndrome), 16
and tricyclic antidepressants, 30, 37*t*

Administration. *See* Dosing/administration

Adrenergic agents, 136–154

Aerosol inhalers, psychiatric side effects of, 167

Aggression
and antipsychotic agents, 83–84
and anxiolytics/sedatives, 126–127
and lithium, 101–102
and propranolol, 147–148

AIDS, 167–171

Akathisia/motor restlessness
as antipsychotic side effect, 88
and beta-blockers, 148
as SSRI side effect, 48–49

Albumin, and protein binding, 9

Albuterol, side effects of, 167*t*

U

Unipolar depression, and lithium, 100–101

V

Valproic acid. *See* Anticonvulsants

Venlafaxine, 57*t*, 63

Volume of distribution (V_d), of drug, 8–9

W

Wellbutrin. *See* Bupropion

Wilson's Disease, 162

Withdrawal dyskinesia, as antipsychotic side effect, 88–89